TRUST MATTERS IN HEALTHCARE

STATE OF HEALTH SERIES

Edited by Chris Ham, Professor of Health Policy and Management at the University of Birmingham and Director of the Strategy Unit at the Department of Health.

Current and forthcoming titles

TRUST MATTERS IN HEALTHCARE

Michael Calnan and Rosemary Rowe

 Open University Press

Open University Press
McGraw-Hill Education
McGraw-Hill House
Shoppenhangers Road
Maidenhead
Berkshire
England
SL6 2QL

email: enquiries@openup.co.uk
world wide web: www.openup.co.uk

and Two Penn Plaza, New York, NY 10121-289, USA

First published 2008

A catalogue record of this book is available from the British Library

ISBN-13: 978 0 335 222834 (pb)   978 0 335 222841 (hb)
ISBN-10: 0 335 22283 8 (pb)   0 335 22284 6 (hb)

Library of Congress Cataloging-in-Publication Data
CIP data has been applied for

Typeset by RefineCatch Limited, Bungay, Suffolk
Printed in Great Britain by Bell and Bain Ltd, Glasgow

Fictitious names of companies, products, people, characters and/or data
that may be used herein (in case studies or in examples) are not intended to
represent any real individual, company, product or event.

The *McGraw·Hill* Companies

To Josie, Lissie and Benji (Calnan) and Sophie and Emily (Rowe)

CONTENTS

SERIES EDITOR'S INTRODUCTION

Health services in many developed countries have come under critical scrutiny in recent years. In part this is because of increasing expenditure, much of it funded from public sources, and the pressure this has put on governments seeking to control public spending. Also important has been the perception that resources allocated to health services are not always deployed in an optimal fashion. Thus at a time when the scope for increasing expenditure is extremely limited, there is a need to search for ways of using existing budgets more efficiently. A further concern has been the desire to ensure access to health care of various groups on an equitable basis. In some countries this has been linked to a wish to enhance patient choice and to make service providers more responsive to patients as consumers.

Underlying these specific concerns are a number of more fundamental developments which have a significant bearing on the performance of health services. Three are worth highlighting. First, there are demographic changes, including the ageing population and the decline in the proportion of the population of working age. These changes will both increase the demand for health care and at the same time limit the ability of health services to respond to this demand.

Second, advances in medical science will also give rise to new demands within the health services. These advances cover a range of possibilities, including innovations in surgery, drug therapy, screening and diagnosis. The pace of innovation quickened as the end of the twentieth century approached, with significant implications for the funding and provision of services.

Third, public expectations of health services are rising as those who use services demand higher standards of care. In part, this is stimulated by developments within the health service, including the availability of new technology. More fundamentally, it stems from the emergence of a more educated and informed population, in which people are accustomed to being treated as consumers rather than patients.

Against this background, policy makers in a number of countries are reviewing the future of health services. Those countries which have traditionally relied on a market in health care are making greater use of regulation and planning. Equally, those countries which have traditionally relied on regulation and planning are moving towards a more competitive approach. In no country is there complete satisfaction with existing methods of financing and delivery, and everywhere there is a search for new policy instruments.

The aim of this series is to contribute to debate about the future of health services through an analysis of major issues in health policy. These issues have been chosen because they are both of current interest and of enduring importance. The series is intended to be accessible to students and informed lay readers as well as to specialists working in this field. The aim is to go beyond a textbook approach to health policy analysis and to encourage authors to move debate about their issues forward. In this sense, each book presents a summary of current research and thinking, and an exploration of future policy directions.

Professor Chris Ham
Professor of Health Policy and Management at the University of Birmingham

PREFACE

Trust in health care is an important, topical and rich area for research and there is a growing interest in these issues within academic, policy and practitioner circles. This book attempts to consider at least some of the salient questions in this field. It is based on a programme of research (2002–2007) carried out by the authors while they worked at the Medical Research Councils' Health Services Research Collaboration, which was based in the Department of Social Medicine at the University of Bristol. It began through our involvement with an international study coordinated by NIVEL in Utrecht in The Netherlands, which was exploring the relationship between different types of healthcare system (NHS compared with Social Insurance and so on) and levels of public trust.

We carried out the national survey in England and Wales. Some of the evidence from this national survey and the international survey is reported in Chapter 1 but as with many of these large and broad-scale surveys, they tend to raise more questions than they answer. The analysis of the survey data particularly raised issues about the conceptualization of trust and confidence, the relationship between interpersonal and institutional trust, and the salience and meaning of trust to different groups living in different circumstances with different types of illness. These appeared, at least at face value, fruitful areas for research but we decided that we needed to carry out a comprehensive review of the empirical research, as well as looking at the theoretical and policy literature before deciding on which specific topic we should focus our interest. The product of this review was 'An agenda for research into Trust in Healthcare', which was presented at a special Nuffield Trust seminar, and these ideas were subsequently developed in an international workshop that focused on the theoretical and methodological challenges. The seminar and workshop identified a range of questions that need to be addressed in research. Some of the research questions on this agenda have been explored in the national survey that formed part of an international comparison. The qualitative study, which also draws on this agenda and is the major focus in this book, explores trust relations between patients, practitioners, and managers in two different clinical and organizational settings, that is type 2 diabetes in primary care and hip surgery in secondary care. This study looks at the meaning and salience of trust to patients, practitioners and managers and how it is built, sustained and broken. Our study, as will become evident, only scratches the surface of the research that needs to be carried out in this area but the hope is that the reader will share our view that trust relations really do matter to patients, healthcare practitioners, and health service managers.

ACKNOWLEDGEMENTS

We carried out the major part of the data collection and analysis of the qualitative interview data ourselves but our thanks go to Dimtirios Spyridinidios for his help with the interviews with the hip patients and to Katrina Ford and Gwen Coombs for their clerical and administrative support throughout the many phases of the research. Thanks also go to Professor Ian Learmonth for his support in setting up the hip case study and to Dr Colin Dayan for his help with the diabetes case study. We are indebted to all the informants, patients, practitioners and managers from the two trusts and the practice who gave up their valuable time to be interviewed. Finally, we would like to thank Professor Paul Dieppe, then the Director of the MRC HSRC, for his support and encouragement throughout the research. This research was funded by the MRC HSRC and the Nuffield Trust.

Michael Calnan and Rosemary Rowe
January 2008

1

TRUST IN THE CONTEXT OF HEALTHCARE

The aim of this introductory chapter is to provide a rationale for examining trust in healthcare and a context for the different elements of trust examined in the following chapters. Definitions of trust are outlined and explored along with a discussion of some of the elements of trust which may be particularly important in the context of the provision of healthcare. First, however, it is important to consider broader discourses of trust, in which debates regarding trust specifically in healthcare are set, and in which there is currently a tendency to portray trust as a declining commodity, under threat from globalization and social change.

THE DECLINE IN TRUST: A DISCOURSE

The concept of trust appears to have become the focus of renewed interest both from academics and policy makers primarily because it is believed that existing bases of social collaboration and agreement are under threat or have been eroded (Misztal 1996). This is claimed to be a product of the increasing uncertainties associated with reflexivity, globalization and risk which are believed to be characteristic of high or late modernity (Giddens 1990; Beck 1992). This, according to Scambler and Britten (2001) has led to commentators emphasizing: 'the significance of trust for post-fordist economics activities, for the invigoration of civil society and for face-to-face relations with friends, lovers and family' (Scambler and Britten 2001: 58).

Trust, as will be shown, is fundamental in the provision of healthcare but according to some writers it too has not been immune from these wider social changes, with trust in doctors and in the medical profession under threat from a number of different sources (Scambler and Britten 2001). The first of these is the rise in consumerism and the shift from organized to disorganized capitalism which has led to the so-called culture of 'shopping around' and cultural pluralism which has permeated the use of healthcare. The second concerns the shift towards a post-modern culture in which science, including biomedicine, has been deprivileged with active trust and citizenship becoming a more common feature of critical modern reasoning and professional expertise becoming increasingly contested. This is linked with the third concern; that is the decline in the status of modern medicine, which is witnessed by the discussion of the processes of deprofessionalism and proletarianization and the attendant threats to the cultural authority and clinical and economic autonomy of doctors. Finally, there is the marketization of healthcare and the more direct or overt link between financial and clinical considerations which may raise doubts about the altruistic motives of doctors (Scambler and Britten 2001) who are claimed to be working in the interests of organizations rather than patients. Thus, much of the renewed interest in trust relations in health care has developed in the context of the alleged decline in trust in medicine. These debates will be considered in more detail at a later stage in this book but what we turn to now is why is trust so important in the provision of healthcare?

THE SALIENCE OF TRUST IN HEALTHCARE

Trust appears to be necessary where there is uncertainty and a level of risk (Jones 1998), be it high, moderate or low, and this element of risk appears to be derived from an individual's uncertainty regarding the motives, intentions and future actions of another on whom the individual is reliant (Mayer et al. 1995; Mishra 1996). Thus, the salience of trust will vary from context to context as will the conditions for generating trust (Rose-Ackerman 2001) but it appears to be particularly important in relation to the provision of healthcare because it is a setting which is characterized by uncertainty and an element of risk regarding the competence and intentions of the practitioner on whom the patient is reliant (Titmuss 1968; Alaszeski 2003). For example, Titmuss (1987) suggests that the unique features of healthcare derive primarily from the prevalence of uncertainty and unpredictability and lists 13 distinctive characteristics that pervade modern health care systems. The need for interpersonal trust relates to the vulnerability associated with being ill as well as the information asymmetries and unequal relationships which arise from the specialist nature of scientific medical knowledge (Calnan et al. 2004) as well as the social position of the medical profession. Scientific medicines' expertise or claims to expertise appears to be the basic condition for generating trust in this context (Rose-Ackerman 2001) although the affective component may also have an influence (Hall et al. 2001).

Trust will probably be salient to healthcare irrespective of the system which provides it because of the uncertainty and unpredictability which characterizes it. However, in the UK NHS trust has traditionally played an important part in the relationship between its three key actors: the state, healthcare practitioners, and patients and the public. The arrangements, at least in the 'old' NHS, were that service users were to trust the judgement, knowledge and expertise of health professionals to provide a competent service which met their needs and they were to trust the state to ensure equity in the allocation of public goods and services. Thus, in the NHS we can distinguish between trust relations at the micro level between an individual patient and clinician, between one clinician and another or between a clinician and a manager, and those at the macro level, which include patient and public trust in clinicians and managers in general, in a particular healthcare organization, and in the NHS as a healthcare system and institution.

The former are broadly categorized as interpersonal and organizational trust relations while the latter constitute different types of institutional trust (see Figure 1.1). This simple classification of the different types of trust relationships will provide the framework for the theoretical and empirical analysis presented in the following chapters. This analysis should shed further light on the possible relationship between these different types of trust and whether other forms of trust relationship not covered by this classification are important in the context of healthcare provision.

A review of the literature of trust relations in healthcare (Calnan and Rowe 2004) highlighted that most empirical research has been mainly carried out in the USA where there is a more explicit link between economic incentives and clinical practice, and the consequent dangers of supplier-induced demand, and where trust in the altruism of doctors' motives is not a given (see Figure 1.2).

However Hall (2006) suggests a number of other reasons for this focus. First, it might reflect the 'sanctity' of the personal relationship that patients in the USA have with their freely chosen physicians.

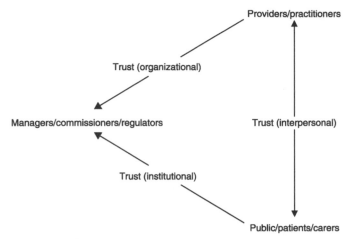

Figure 1.1   Framing trust relationships in health care
Source: Calnan and Rowe (2006).

Second, according to Hall (2006) the commercialization and the privatization of US medicine has led to the demand for the development of comparative performance indicators for evaluating providers so that US consumers can be more knowledgeable about what they are paying for. An interest in the USA in trust research has also

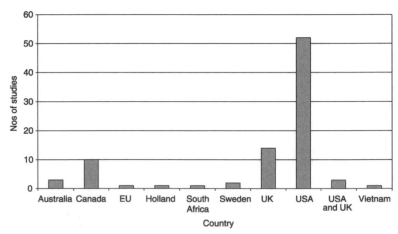

Figure 1.2   Research into trust by country
Source: Calnan and Rowe (2004).

̱emmed (Hall 2006) from the perceived threat of managed care ̱ the doctor–patient relationship. Trust in medicine was implicit but this changed as a result of concern that trust and the quality of the doctor–patient relationship may have been undermined by managed care insurance such as financial incentives to withhold care, restricted choice of doctors, and insurers' oversight of doctors.

This research has addressed threats to patient–provider relationships although trust in healthcare systems from the patient's perspective, at least in the USA, has been neglected. Hall (2006: 457) accounts for this neglect in terms of the highly fragmented and disorganized nature of the US health system 'simply put, we have not put much effort into studying our system because there is no system'. Studies in the organizational literature, which is also still in short supply, suggest that trust relations in the workforce, between providers and between providers and managers, may also influence patient–provider relationships and levels of trust (Gilson et al. 2005). This approach suggests that trust is not primarily dispositional or an individual attribute or psychological state, but is constructed from a set of interpersonal behaviours or from a shared identity. These behaviours are underpinned by sets of institutional rules, laws and customs (Rowe 2003; Gilson 2006).

Research into trust has been conducted from a variety of disciplinary perspectives. Studies in social psychology and economics have tended to focus on the attributes of the trustor (beliefs about or calculations of trustees' motives; past experiences of healthcare and providers) and the characteristics of the trustee (their ability, competence, benevolence, integrity, reputation and communication skills). Taking the rational choice economics approach, trust may be reduced to instrumental risk assessment by individual actors, that is a rational gamble that the personal gains from trusting will outweigh the risks and costs involved. For example, an economic analysis of why the public place trust in voluntary associations (Anheier and Kendall 2002) suggests that voluntary associations are run by those who have a stake in services provided to meet their needs and because they are non-profit-making and less likely to exploit user vulnerability. However, this ignores how trust may be constructed through the use of myths, images and other symbolic constructions. For example, Newman (1998) points to the use of informal social mechanisms such as gossip to communicate information through organizations, in the process contributing to the creation of trust and distrust. In this sense trust may be manufactured by the construction or manipulation of images rather than consideration of rational self-interest.

The sociological literature stresses that theoretical models must also consider contextual factors: the organizational context; the stakes involved; the balance of power within the relationship; the perception of the level of risk; and the alternatives available to the trustor (Luhmann 1979; Barber 1983; Zucker 1986; Mayer et al. 1995; Tyler and Kramer 1996). In this book we take a predominantly sociological approach, seeking to understand how the meaning and enactment of trust is influenced both by the micro- and macro-social context and in particular how changes in the organization and delivery of healthcare as well as broader social changes may have affected trust relations in the UK NHS.

TRUST AND ITS CONSTRUCTION

Trust has been characterized as a multilayered concept primarily consisting of a cognitive element (grounded on rational and instrumental judgements) and an affective dimension (grounded on relationships and affective bonds generated through interaction, empathy and identification with others) (Rempel et al. 1975; Lewis and Weigert 1985; Mayer et al. 1995; Lewicki and Bunker 1996; Gambetta 1988; Gilson 2003). Trust appears to be necessary where there is uncertainty regarding the motives, intentions and future actions of another on whom the individual is dependent (Mayer et al. 1995; Mishra 1996). Luhmann (1979: 8) suggests that trust is necessary for us as it increases tolerance of uncertainty; trust 'reduces social complexity by going beyond available information and generalizing expectations of behaviour in that it replaces missing information with an internally guaranteed security'. In this respect it is enabling as it encourages people to take risks when the outcomes are uncertain. Trust may vary in terms of its quality and quantity. For example, in elaborating on the nature of social capital (Putnam 2000) makes a distinction between 'thick' trust associated with close family relationships and 'thin' trust for more casual contacts. It is important to identify what people trust others to do as much as how much trust they have. For example, patients may have a lot of trust in nurses to monitor their long-term condition but trust them less when managing their medication. Misztal (1996) proposes a sociological approach to trust based on three assumptions. The first of these is that trust should be understood in terms of its functions for social order which relate to stability, cohesion and collaboration. The second assumption is that trust requires ontological security and conditions under which social bonds can be promoted. The third assumption is that trust has a role as a social good or social capital.

In the context of healthcare, the most prevalent elements include confidence in competence (skill and knowledge), as well as whether the trustee is working in the best interests of the trustor. The latter tends to cover honesty, confidentiality and caring, and showing respect (Mechanic and Meyer 2000; Hall et al. 2001) whereas the former may include both technical and social/communication skills although the relative importance of these skills may depend on the organizational setting in which the care is provided. The vulnerability associated with being ill may specifically lead trust in the context of medical settings to have a stronger emotional and instinctive component (Coulson 1998; Hall et al. 2001). Trust relationships have therefore been characterized by one party, the trustor, having positive expectations regarding both the competence of the other party (competence trust), the trustee, and that they will work in their best interests (intentional trust). For example, as Davies (1999) suggests, all definitions of trust embody the notion of expectations: expectations by the public that healthcare providers will demonstrate knowledge, skill and competence: further expectations too that they will behave as true agents (that is, in the patient's best interests) and with beneficence, fairness and integrity. It is these collective expectations that form the basis of trust.

However, for some writers (Giddens 1991) these trust relations are built on symbolic signs of expertise rather than altruistic principles and intentions and actual performance. Barbalet (2005) suggests that trust works as a 'tranquillizer' in social relations in which trust shuts down the trust giver's uncertainty in the face of the trust takers' freedom to act how they wish. Yet, the general point that these two writers allude to is that trust must be seen and understood within the context in which the relationships take place. This involves making explicit the social and cultural assumptions and expectations which are embedded in and emerge from these contexts. This is believed to be relevant to both interpersonal and institutional trust relationships (Gilson 2006). For example, Greener (2003), drawing on Luke's three faces of power, has developed a power-focused taxonomy of trust which illustrates the influence of overt and covert forms of power. Greener's first category of trust is voluntary which is characterized by an absence of calculation and the presence of mutual or shared trust such as in friendship. This can be manifest in interpersonal relations where there is a mutual understanding and a shared identity which might develop and be built up in a doctor–patient relationship over time, possibly in the context of chronic illness. It could also be manifest in trust in an institution such as public confidence in the NHS because of its reputation or through evidence from more visible performance information and trust in healthcare practitioners because of their standard of professional training. The second category of trust is involuntary where trust is forced on someone as there is no alternative and dependency or reliance is enforced. It is contingent on and constrained by power relations at either the interpersonal or institutional levels. This is manifest in the provision of healthcare by the power relations brought about, at least in part, by the asymmetries in clinical and system knowledge in the provider–patient relationship and the prevalence of uncertainty previously described by Titmuss (1987). Greener's (2003) third category of trust is hegemonic which involves an unquestioning acceptance and subservience to a system such as the inherent trust in the NHS general practitioner system which led to a doctor such as Harold Shipman being trusted unconditionally.

The trust literature makes little explicit mention of risk, other than in relation to vulnerability (Connell and Mannion 2006). However, for many writers the concepts of trust and risk are closely related. For example, Jones (1998) in a philosophical review identifies risk as one of the key elements that should be accommodated in accounts of trust as trust involves risk because those who trust run the risk of letting those they trust near things that they care about (Jones 1998). The trustee may be unaware of or choose not to be aware of the risks such as in the case of blind trust. However, trust is not simply a vague or optimistic hope and does not require a denial of all risk (Jones 1998). For example, as Entwistle and Quick (2006: 407) argue when writing about trust in the context of patient safety, '. . . we should also accept that the placing of trust by a patient in a healthcare provider does not necessarily depend on the patient being ignorant of healthcare safety problems, being convinced that their healthcare providers have exceptional safety records (or prospects) or being totally convinced that no harm will befall them'.

DOES TRUST MATTER?

The case for examining trust in healthcare tends to hinge upon theoretical arguments sometimes complemented by empirical evidence. At the level of interpersonal trust between patient and practitioner, it has been argued that trust is important for its potential therapeutic effects (Mechanic 1998) although evidence to support such claims is still in short supply mainly because of the lack of intervention studies or quasi-experimental studies (see Figure 1.3) examining the effect of trust on health outcomes (Calnan and Rowe 2004). However, there is a considerable body of evidence that shows trust appears to mediate therapeutic processes and has an indirect influence on health outcomes through its impact on patient satisfaction, adherence to treatment and continuity with a provider, and that it encourages patients to access healthcare and to make appropriate disclosure of information so that accurate and timely diagnosis can be made (Calnan and Rowe 2004). For example, the importance of trust to the quality of doctor–patient interactions emerged spontaneously in a number of studies investigating patients' experience of healthcare (Thorne and Robinson 1988; Safran et al. 2001; Goold and Klipp 2002; Lings et al. 2003; Trojan and Yonge 2003) with trust in doctors' expertise a key concern for breast cancer patients in the UK (Burkitt Wright et al. 2004) and AIDS patients in the USA (Carr 2001).

Trust appears to mediate therapeutic processes; higher levels of trust have been associated with acceptance of recommended treatment (Paul and Oyebode 1999; McKneally and Martin 2000; Altice et al. 2001; Collins et al. 2002; Hall et al. 2002; Stapleton et al. 2002; Dibben and Lena, 2003; Jackson et al. 2004), lower treatment anxiety (Caterinicchio 1979) and adherence to treatment (Safran et al. 1998; Mosley-Williams et al. 2002; Thom et al. 2002; Lukoschek 2003).

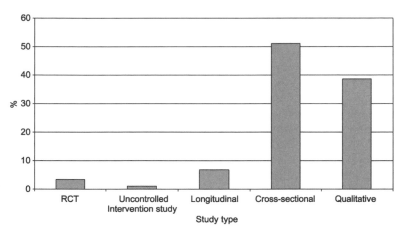

Figure 1.3 Types of studies researching trust
Source: Calnan and Rowe (2004).

For patients with mental illness trust facilitated disclosure (Repper et al. 1994) and helped them to take control of their mental health (Kai and Crosland 2001; Svedberg et al. 2003), although it did not appear to moderate response to psychotherapy (McKay et al. 1997). Studies also suggest that trust facilitates access to health services (Cooper-Patrick et al. 1997; Sharma et al. 2003; Matthews et al. 2004) and the acceptance and use of new vaccines by patients (Rothstein 1998).

Trust also appears to matter to patients as well as healthcare providers. In a number of studies investigating patients' experience of healthcare, trust emerged spontaneously as a quality indicator, with patients suggesting that high-quality doctor–patient interactions are characterized by high levels of trust, for example see Safran et al. (1998). Trust, although highly correlated with patient satisfaction (Thom and Ribisi 1999), is believed to be a distinct concept. Trust is forward looking and reflects an attitude to a new or ongoing relationship whereas satisfaction tends to be based on past experience and refers to assessment of providers' performance. It has been suggested that trust is a more sensitive indicator of performance than patient satisfaction (Thom et al. 2004) and might be used as a potential 'marker' for how patients evaluate the quality of healthcare. In addition, several studies suggest that trust levels have been associated with patients' loyalty to their provider (Arksey and Sloper 1999; Safran et al. 2001; Keating et al. 2002;) and their evaluation of and willingness to recommend hospitals and medical care (Caterinicchio 1979; Joffe et al., 2003).

In contrast to the sizeable literature assessing trust from the patient perspective, studies examining either the value and impact of trust from the practitioner perspective and from a managerial or organizational perspective are very limited (see Figures 1.4 and 1.5).

From an organizational perspective trust is believed to be important in its own right: it is intrinsically important for the provision of effective healthcare and has even been described as a collective good, like social trust or social capital (Khodyakov 2007). Specific organizational benefits that might be derived from trust as a form of social capital include the reduction in transaction costs due to lower surveillance and monitoring and the general enhancement of efficiency (Gilson 2003).

In terms of the provider's perspective, trust has also been identified as being necessary for the uptake of evidence-based medicine by Canadian family physicians and could change the amount of

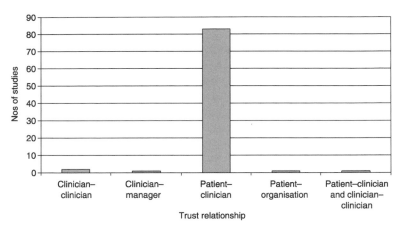

Figure 1.4 Focus of studies identified in literature review
Source: Calnan and Rowe (2004).

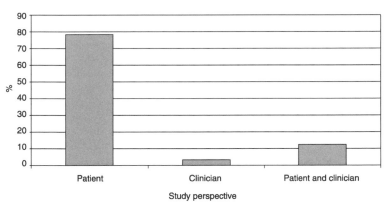

Figure 1.5 Perspective of interest in studies in literature review
Source: Calnan and Rowe (2004).

time spent with patients (Jackson et al. 2004). In studies that considered the impact of trust on workplace relations in healthcare settings, trust facilitated commitment to the organization (Laschinger et al. 2000), encouraged collaborative practice between clinicians (Hallas et al. 2004), was associated with job satisfaction and motivation (Gilson et al. 2005), and where trust was low nurses spent more time assessing the communication behaviour of other nurses (Northouse 1979).

A further broader potential benefit of why trust matters to health-care systems has been identified by Gilson (2006) who suggests that a health system based on trusting relationships can contribute to generating wider social value. This argument is based on the understanding that health systems do not just produce healthcare and have the goal of improving health. In addition, as with other social and political institutions, they establish the social norms that shape human behaviour and so act as a repository and producer of wider social value. To the extent that these norms help establish a moral community whom you can trust, they may provide the basis for generalized trust (Gilson 2006).

In summary, there is substantial empirical evidence that trust mediates healthcare processes, but no direct evidence of a beneficial therapeutic effect on health outcomes. It appears to be a key indicator of the quality of clinician–patient relations and patients have identified it as a marker for how they evaluate their experience of healthcare. Little is known about the impact of trust in clinician–manager relations and between clinicians on organizational and clinical performance and on patient–clinician relations.

THE 'DARK SIDE' OF TRUST

What are the costs, dangers or the 'dark side' of trust? Gilson (2006) identifies at least three from the theoretical literature. The first is associated with shared identity which allows the development of a particularized form of trust that enables cooperation in pursuit of morally unworthy acts. She illustrates this through the activities of organizations such as the Mafia. Second, there is the abuse of power on the basis of trust which she sees as a widespread danger (Warren 1999) and as trust usually involves an asymmetrical relationship between trustor, trustee and a valued good, it sets up a potential power relation. Trust may provide legitimacy for the exercise of power but 'blind trust' without caution may also enable the abuse of power, in the form of exploitation or domination. The third and associated danger for healthcare is the vulnerability of patients from 'deprived' circumstances (Gilson 2006). For example, the consequences of misplaced trust can, particularly for groups living in poverty, threaten livelihoods and lives (Coulson 1998) and it may be easier to trust and take risks if you are powerful and wealthy. Similarly, wealthy as opposed to poorer people may be seen to be more likely to be trustworthy and less of a risk to 'invest' in. Thus, Gilson (2006) argues that the poor may be further marginalized as a result of trust relations. Connell and Mannion (2006) explore this theme further by speculating on the negative aspects of high trust cultures in organizations. They suggest that trust may be difficult, costly and time consuming to create but once established may be easily lost through inappropriate actions. In addition, high *trust* cultures may offer the opportunity to exploit the lack of vigilance and assessment of performance and cosy relationships may stifle innovation and foster corrupt practice and exclusivity. Thus, given the potential benefits and costs of trusting relationships, there may be a need to explore what levels and forms of trust contribute to positive health outcomes and healthcare performance and what levels of distrust maybe necessary to counter the abuse of power (Gilson 2006).

RESEARCHING TRUST RELATIONS

Empirical research into trust relations (Calnan and Rowe 2004) has tended to explore: the nature and form of trust in terms of its different dimensions and types; levels of trust; the factors that build, sustain or detract from trust; and the effects of high or low trust.

The nature and form of trust: empirical evidence

Studies have investigated the nature and form of trust, either through qualitative research to understand patients' understanding of the concept or through the development of instruments to measure trust. A number of scales measuring different trust relations (public trust in healthcare, trust in a particular physician, trust in the medical profession generally, and distrust in the healthcare system) have been developed that have been found to have high internal consistency and which are available for use in future studies (Hall 2006).

Qualitative research which has explored patients' understanding of the concept of trust is limited but those studies which have done so have identified different types of trust. Dibben and Lena's (2003) study of patients attending nutrition clinics found that doctors sought to establish 'swift trust' early in the consultation by identifying areas of agreement and shared experience as the six monthly interval between consultations prevented frequent interaction and the development of trust over time. Lee-Treweek (2002) found that patients relied upon 'network trust' (the views of trusted family, friends or colleagues) in order to initially attend an osteopathic practice but that thereafter 'experiential trust' ensured their continued attendance. Thorne and Robinson's (1989) study of patients with chronic illness distinguished between the 'naive trust' typical of the start of clinician–patient relations and 'reconstructed trust', trust which was re-established by patients after experiencing a period of disenchantment with their provider. The extent and way in which trust was reconstructed affected the type of clinician–patient relationship, varying from 'hero worship' when trust was re-established by designating an individual healthcare professional distinct from all others to trust, to 'resignation' when there was little evidence of any trust. Sobo's (2001) study emphasized that trust has a non-rational dimension, anchored by patient dependence and hope. It is of note that all the qualitative studies which have explored conceptual understanding of trust have done so solely from the patient's perspective and it is not known whether clinical and managerial perspectives on trust vary significantly from patients' views.

Levels of trust

A considerable number of studies, using cross-sectional designs and mainly conducted in the USA, have investigated levels of patient and public trust in clinicians, the health system, or health insurers. There is little empirical evidence that patients' trust in health professionals has eroded in recent years, with trust in clinicians in all countries remaining high. In the USA Joffe et al.'s (2003) large survey of patients discharged from hospitals in Massachusetts reported that 77 per cent always trusted nurses and 87 per cent always trusted doctors, and Mainous et al. (2004) found in their study that most cancer patients had similarly high levels of trust. Levels of trust may, however, vary according to the type of illness, extent of risk, and the patient's experience of medical care. Although Mechanic and Meyer's (2000) qualitative study did not use measures of trust levels, it was evident from patient narratives that these varied according to their type of illness. Patients with breast cancer appeared to have the highest level of trust, in part because the life-threatening nature of the disease made it more important for them to feel they could trust their physicians. In contrast, Lyme disease sufferers who had experienced difficulties in obtaining a diagnosis and treatment talked much more about loss of trust.

The impact of managed care on levels of trust appears to be mixed. While HMO members have less trust in doctors as a group than in their own doctor (Goold and Klipp 2002), (which supports

Hall et al.'s (2002) finding that interpersonal trust is on average 25 per cent higher than general trust), 85 per cent of members trusted their doctor all or most of the time (Grumbach et al. 1999) with similar high levels reported by members in another HMO, irrespective of the type of provider payment (Kao et al. 1998a). In contrast, Haas et al. (2003) reported that in US communities with more than 50 per cent managed care, individuals were less likely to trust their doctor to put their medical needs first, and young physicians in the USA considered that trust in them had diminished over the past five years (Sulmasy et al. 2000). Haas' study comprised a survey of US households and it may be that lower levels of trust are reported when members of the public rather than patients are questioned: that while patient trust in clinicians remains high, public trust has fallen. In a rare longitudinal study assessing changes in levels of trust, Murphy et al. (2001) reported that trust in doctors among Massachusetts employees of a public sector organization had significantly declined between 1996–1999.

In Canada patients from breast cancer, prostate cancer and fracture clinics had varying levels of trust in clinicians: 36.1 per cent reported high trust and 48.6 per cent reported moderate trust with only 9.0 per cent having low trust (Kraetschner et al. 2004). As in the USA, patients have lower trust in the medical system generally and trust in policy actors may fall to particularly low levels during times of change to the healthcare system (Kehoe and Ponting 2003). Given the uncertain impact of managed care in the USA it is interesting that in a comparison of the USA and the UK, Mainous et al. (2001) found no significant difference in the levels of trust of patients in their family physicians; both were high (more than 44 points on a scale that ranges from 11 to 55). Hall (2006) offers a number of possible explanations for the higher levels of trust that US patients and/or members of the public express in individuals as opposed to medical institutions. First, people typically have stronger trust in individuals than in professional systems or organizations. Second, people are generally inclined to have an optimistic view of themselves and their personal relationships. This is particularly important in the context of healthcare because of the patients' position of vulnerability. Third, it could be a methodological artefact, reflecting a form of cognitive adjustment or social desirability bias in response to questions about trust (patients may have good reasons for not being overtly critical of their doctor). Finally, trust in individual health professionals may have a stronger affective component than trust in healthcare organizations, which may reflect a more critical evaluation and a greater emphasis on the cognitive element of trust.

Little empirical research has been conducted to investigate the nature of trust relations within the UK health system; instead most studies have focused on assessing levels of trust. These studies confirm the familiar pattern that suggests that while patients retain high levels of trust in individual clinicians ('your own doctor') (Calnan and Williams 1992; Mainous et al. 2001; Tarrant et al. 2003; Calnan and Sanford 2004), lower levels of trust are found for healthcare institutions. For example, evidence from a recent postal survey (n = 1187) (Calnan and Sanford 2004), carried out in 2002/3, on a random sample of people (18+) living in England and Wales, showed that 76 per cent reported that they always or most of the time trusted NHS hospital doctors to put the interests of their patients above the convenience of the hospital (see Figure 1.6). The comparable figure for hospital nurses was 85 per cent, for general practitioners 83 per cent, and for general practice nurses 87 per cent. Similarly, when asked about levels of confidence in different healthcare practitioners, 89 per cent said that they either had a fair or a great deal of confidence in general practitioners, 87 per cent in hospital doctors, and 89 per cent in nurses.[1]

The reported average level of confidence and trust in today's healthcare system was 6 out of a score of 10 and this declined to 5.6 when respondents in this survey were asked about confidence and trust in the healthcare system of the future. This lower level of trust in the healthcare system as an institution seems to be reflected in the

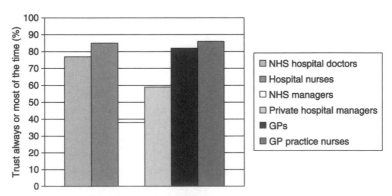

Figure 1.6 Levels of trust in health services staff: putting interests of patients above convenience of organizations

Source: Calnan and Rowe (2006).

levels of trust shown in health services managers. The survey evidence showed only 29 per cent reporting that they had a great deal of confidence (3 per cent) or a fair amount of confidence (26 per cent) in health service managers. Private hospital managers fared better than NHS hospital managers in that 59 per cent said that they think private hospital managers would always, or most of the time, put the interests of their patients above the convenience of the hospital compared with 38 per cent of NHS managers (see Figure 1.6).

This lower trust in health service managers also appears to be explained by responses to items about trust in specific aspects of the service. The lowest level of trust was found in relation to the performance of the system, that is 75 per cent said that they had little or very little trust in waiting times never being too long. The percentage for 'cost-cutting does not disadvantage patients' was 68 and for 'patients won't be the victims of rising costs of health care' was 70. How important is this lower level of trust in aspects of the performance of the health system? The answer is that it has limited importance, at least according to results of the statistical analysis which explored the determinants of public assessments of confidence in today's NHS care. This survey used 32 specific items measuring six different aspects of the process of healthcare: (a) patient-centered care; (b) macro-level performance and patient care; (c) professional competence; (d) quality of care; (e) communication and provision of information; and (f) quality of cooperation between healthcare providers/practitioners. Top of the league for explaining trust were whether patients are taken seriously and whether they are given enough attention (that is aspects of patient-centered care) followed by items assessing professional expertise ('patients will always get the best treatment' and 'doctors always make the right diagnosis'). The bottom six predictors in the league table mainly consisted of items measuring aspects of macro-level performance such as waiting lists, waiting times and cost-cutting (see Figures 1.7 and 1.8; Tables 1.1 and 1.2).

The results of this statistical analysis suggest that the relationships between the perceived performance of the healthcare system at the macro level and the perceived quality of healthcare provision at the macro level is a complicated one. Research needs to examine how if, in any way, institutional trust influences interpersonal trust and/or vice versa and also on what basis the public and patients assess levels of trust and confidence in health service managers compared with healthcare practitioners. There is evidence of a decrease

Table 1.1   Specific determinants of overall rating of trust/confidence – top six

Rank order	Individual determinants	N	Mean change in overall trust rating per unit lost in trust in individual determinant	95 % CI	p	R^2
27	F: Patients are not given conflicting information	1140	−0.383	(−0.48, −0.29)	0.00	0.05
28	Patients will show doctors respect	1143	−0.376	(−0.48, −0.27)	0.00	0.04
29	B: Waiting times are never too long	1137	−0.358	(−0.45, −0.27)	0.00	0.05
30	B: Cost-cutting does not disadvantage patients	1135	−0.343	(−0.43, −0.26)	0.00	0.05
31	F: High levels of specialization do not cause problems in the healthcare system	1129	−0.278	(−0.38, −0.18)	0.00	0.02
32	B: Patients will be able to pay for their own healthcare if they have to	1128	−0.081	(−0.18, −0.15)	0.10	0.01

Source: Calnan and Rowe 2006.

in satisfaction with the NHS over the last decade or so (Appleby and Rosete 2003) but there is no evidence available about whether there has been a parallel decline in public trust. However, evidence from a Dutch consumer panel survey (van der Schee et al. 2006), which monitored public trust in healthcare in the Netherlands over an eight-year period from 1997 to 2004 showed overall levels remained quite stable. This was in spite of marked changes in healthcare policy during this period along with intense media coverage of public and political discontent about these policy changes. There were some minor fluctuations and, for example, trust in medical specialists

Table 1.2 Specific determinants of overall rating of trust/confidence –
bottom six

Rank order	Individual determinants	N	Mean change in overall trust rating per unit lost in trust in individual determinant	95% CI	p	R^2
1	A: Patients are taken seriously	1140	−0.801	(−0.89, −0.71)	0.00	0.21
2	A: Patients get enough attention	1140	−0.742	(−0.82, −0.66)	0.00	0.21
3	D: Patients will always get the best treatment	1141	−0.703	(−0.78, −0.62)	0.00	0.21
4	D: Doctors always make the right diagnosis	1144	−0.687	(−0.78, −0.59)	0.00	0.16
5	A: Doctors provide their patients with good guidance	1137	−0.651	(−0.74, −0.56)	0.00	0.15
6	F: Healthcare providers are good at cooperating with each other	1136	−0.635	(−0.72, −0.55)	0.00	0.15

Source: Calnan and Rowe (2006).

displayed an upward trend but, overall, general practitioners and specialists are highly trusted by the Dutch public. This pattern of results led the authors to raise doubts about whether trust should be regarded as a strong reflective indicator or predictor of healthcare performance.

With the development of instruments to measure trust in healthcare systems, several studies have reported such data (Straten et al. 2002). For example, there is evidence from an international study using the same core questions and comparing levels of public trust in

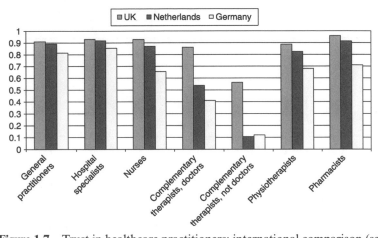

Figure 1.7   Trust in healthcare practitioners: international comparison (see van der Schee et al. 2003)

Source: Calnan and Rowe (2006).

different countries (England and Wales, Germany and the Netherlands) with different healthcare systems (van der Schee et al. 2003). Results showed that levels of trust in different healthcare practitioners were higher in England and Wales than in the other two countries. However, for different aspects of healthcare, levels of trust in Germany were consistently marked lower than in the other two countries.

The authors postulated four possible influences on variations in public trust in healthcare systems. Two of these characteristics are associated with the healthcare system itself; these are the extent and nature of institutional guarantees (for example extent of regulation and protection of patients' rights) and the quality of care provided. The two others were media images, which can be positive and negative (the media tends to amplify a scandal on the one hand and ignore success stories on the other), and the influences of different cultural differences in public attitudes, that is people in different countries may differ in their general orientation or predisposition to trust institutions and people. The authors tentatively conclude that differences in public trust may strongly reflect cultural differences, which clearly affects the applicability of the concept of public trust in international comparisons of healthcare performance (van der Schee et al. 2007).

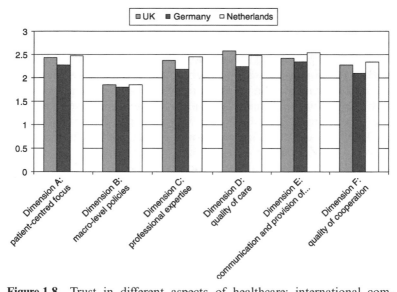

Figure 1.8   Trust in different aspects of healthcare: international comparison

Source: Calnan and Rowe (2006).

In summary, levels of patient trust in specific clinicians appear to continue to be high but there is lower public trust in clinicians in general and healthcare systems. Given the lack of longitudinal studies it is not possible to state whether this marks an erosion of trust, although evidence from regular national surveys in the UK shows an overall decline in public satisfaction (not necessarily trust) with the NHS which is believed to be paralleled in the USA (Mechanic and Schlesinger 1996). However, evidence from the Netherlands shows little change in recent years in levels of public trust in the health system.

The determinants and the development of trust

Given that trust is assumed to be important for an effective therapeutic relationship, it is not surprising that a large proportion of trust research has examined what factors are associated with high levels of trust and how trust can be built and sustained between patients and clinicians. Most of the data are derived from cross-sectional studies; although their findings do not show causal relationships a number of common themes emerge from the research. Most studies emphasize that trust depends on relationship factors more than patient characteristics (Thom et al. 1999; Goold and Klipp 2002; Tarrant et al. 2003; Calnan and Sanford 2004), although others have reported that higher trust levels were found among older, less educated patients (Anderson and Dedrick 1999; Mainous et al. 2001; Balkrishnan et al. 2003; Freburger et al. 2003; Tarrant et al. 2003; Kraetscher et al. in press). A number of studies emphasize that trust can be built if patient views are respected and taken seriously and information is openly shared with patients (Trojan and Yonge 2003; Wilson et al. 1998; Arksey and Sloper 1999; Mechanic and Meyer 2000; Zadoroznyj 2001; Henman et al. 2002; Johansson and Winkvist 2002; Joffe et al. 2003; Burkitt Wright et al. 2004; Mazor et al. 2004). As well as clinicians' interpersonal skills, their technical competence is important for the development of trust (Gibson 1990; Cooper-Patrick et al.1997; Goold and Klipp 2002; Henman et al. 2002; Lee-Treweek 2002; Lings et al. 2003; McKneally and Martin 2000; Thom et al. 2002; Burkitt Wright et al. 2004; Gilson et al. 2005). Zadoroznyj's study of Australian women who have gone through childbirth suggests that if clinicians have good interpersonal skills then their technical competence is secondary in patients' judgement of their trustworthiness.

Several studies have examined the impact of ethnicity on variations in levels of trust in the USA. In a large household survey Doescher (2000) reported that lower levels of trust in doctors were associated with African-Americans compared to white Americans and this finding was confirmed in Boulware et al.'s (2002) survey in Baltimore. However, among African-American patients, as in Mosley-Williams et al.'s (2002) study of lupus sufferers, differences in trust by race disappeared.

The potential impact of managed care on trust has stimulated studies that have investigated the contribution of choice of provider, provider payment method, and continuity of provider to patient trust. The results have been mixed. In a cross-sectional survey choice of provider was associated with higher trust levels (Kao et al. 1998b). But Hsu et al. (2003) conducted an RCT to assess the impact of choice of provider and found that although it increased satisfaction and provider retention it did not significantly increase trust. Kao et al. (1998b) reported that patient knowledge of payment method was not associated with lower levels of trust, possibly because physician behaviour mediates any impact of this knowledge. This was confirmed by Hall et al. (2002) in an RCT – using a letter disclosing payment method with explanatory follow-up call. However, if HMO members experienced difficulties (Keating et al. 2002), such as in accessing a specialist (Grumbach et al. 1999) or if they had sought a second opinion (Hall et al. 2002), this was associated with lower trust.

Other studies have addressed the importance of continuity of provider in building up trust over time as the clinician and patient increase their knowledge and understanding of each other. Kao et al. (1998b) reported that choice of physician and continuity with provider increased trust among HMO members in Atlanta and Mainous et al. (2001), Jackson et al. (2004) and Baker et al. (2003) found that continuity of care was associated with higher levels of trust. Carr's (2001) qualitative study of AIDS patients also found that trust was linked to provider continuity but participants emphasized that trust had to be renegotiated at various points. However, Tarrant et al.'s (2003) study of English patients in primary care found no correlation between trust and continuity, and Caterinicchio (1979) reported that the quality of interaction, not continuity, was important. This was similarly shown in Dibben and Lena's (2003) study where the infrequency of consultations created little opportunity for trust to develop over time; instead doctors sought to build trust by sharing information, identifying areas of common ground and by emphasizing patient self-competence. Thorne and Robinson's research (1988, 1989) with patients suffering from a variety of chronic conditions found that trust in clinicians developed when clinicians showed their trust in patient competence to manage their illness.

More recently studies have addressed the importance of patient participation in decision-making and its contribution to the development of trust between clinician and patient. For some patients trust was linked to the professional status of their clinician and they did not expect an active role in decision-making (Trojan and Yonge 1993; Zadoroznyj 2001; Johansson and Winkvist 2002), Kraetschner et al. (2004) refers to this as 'blind trust'. Both Kai and Crossland's (2001) study of patients with mental illness in the UK and Kraetschrner's (2004) research with cancer patients in Canada report that trust was associated with providing patients with the opportunity to express concerns and discuss and negotiate treatment options. Breast cancer surgeons and oncologists in Canada reported that they found trust facilitated shared decision-making (Charles et al. 2003). But patient participation per se does not necessarily result in higher trust. Krupat et al. (2001) found that trust was associated with value congruence regarding patient participation; patient centredness did not produce higher trust if this did not reflect patient preferences for involvement. In Caress et al.'s (2002) UK study of adults with asthma higher levels of trust were associated with more passive decision-making, which reflects Anderson and Dedrick's (1990) study in the USA that reported that patients with low trust wanted more control in medical interactions. The mixed evidence regarding trust and its association with shared decision-making and the uncertainty as to whether role preference determines trust levels or vice versa indicate that further studies which are not cross-sectional are required.

While there is a substantial literature on factors associated with the development of patient trust in clinicians, research into clinician–clinician and clinician–manager relationships is sparse. In Jackson et al.'s (2004) qualitative study family doctors in Nova Scotia reported that trust between providers developed over time through positive experiences, and Hallas et al.'s (2004) small survey found that open and honest communication was associated with greater trust and mutual respect between paediatric nurse practitioners and US pediatricians. Payne and Clark (2003) reported that systemic factors such as job specification as well as interpersonal variables affected trust levels; similarly, Gilson et al.'s study in South Africa suggested that management style and communication practices may increase workplace trust. These limited studies indicate the need for further research to identify how trust is built between clinicians, between clinicians and managers and how this might affect clinician–patient relations and patient trust in healthcare organizations and systems. Hall et al.'s (2002) survey of HMO members found that system trust could help the development of interpersonal trust, without prior knowledge of the individual clinician, but it is not known how clinician–patient trust affects institutional trust. Medical errors and cost containment are associated with distrust of healthcare systems (Rose et al. 2004) and it appears that system-level trust may be linked to cultural differences (van der Schee et al. 2007), but more research is required to investigate what influences trust in healthcare systems.

FOCUS OF THE RESEARCH: STRUCTURE OF THE BOOK

This introductory chapter has presented a rationale for examining trust relations in healthcare from a patient, professional, organizational and policy perspective. This chapter has clearly shown, despite the considerable body of trust literature in existence, that there are still numerous unanswered questions for theoretical and empirical research (see Calnan and Rowe 2004 for a more detailed research agenda). Trust is a complex concept with multiple domains and potentially different forms but very little research has been conducted to increase our conceptual understanding of trust relationships in healthcare or to develop methodologies for exploring such concepts empirically. Conceptually, there is a need to examine whether trust is still salient to relationships within healthcare and if so whether new forms of trust have developed as a result of the changing organizational structure of medical care and the culture of healthcare delivery. Has, for example, patients' blind trust in healthcare practitioners been replaced by a more conditional, informed trust and if so what does this new form of trust look like and what are its implications for patients, practitioners and managers? What of the trust relationships between health professionals and between healthcare managers and health professionals which have been neglected in research up until now? In addition, there are particular methodological challenges to investigating trust; most notably reported expressions of levels of trust may differ from enacted behaviour. Research is needed to identify what beliefs and behaviour might indicate low or high trust in different organizational settings and in different relationships, between clinicians and patients, between patients and healthcare organizations, between healthcare practitioners, and between practitioners and managers.

The major focus of this book is to explore the nature of trust relations between patients and health professionals, between healthcare professionals, and between clinicians and health service managers. Thus, the aim is to examine in some depth interpersonal trust relations, organizational trust and institutional trust, and if and how they may relate to each other. This is explored through a combination of theoretical analysis and empirical research. The later chapters in this book draw mainly on evidence from a recently completed study using qualitative methods to explore trust relations in different clinical and organizational settings in the NHS in England. This exploratory study compares and contrasts evidence from an analysis of two different clinical and organizational settings: treatment of type 2 diabetes in primary care and provision of elective hip replacements in secondary care. Trust may be particularly pertinent to self-management by patients with diabetes as patients need to play an active part in care management and thus are required to develop the necessary levels of competence and motivation for self-management (Skinner and Hampson 2001). Thus, the provider–patient relationship might be characterized by a need for mutual trust with the patient trusting the provider to have the expertise and to provide care and support when required and the provider trusting the patient to develop the expertise and take responsibility for self-care. This case study provides the opportunity to examine how trust operates in the primary care setting and specifically how trust in a particular GP or practice nurse translates into trust in primary care generally and the wider NHS. In acute settings, which are characterized by greater levels of uncertainty and risk, patients' higher dependence on their practitioners may require high levels of trust, and less need for mutual trust. This case study examines how trust operates in an acute setting and how trust in specific hospital clinicians translates into trust in the particular hospital and the wider NHS. The case studies also differ in the potential for patient self-management (greater for diabetes patients) and the extent of patient choice (potentially more salient to patients requiring hip replacements). (For full details of the methodology used see Appendix).

Before this empirical evidence is presented, there is a need to outline and discuss the theoretical perspective taken in this research and this is addressed in Chapter 2 which examines how and why trust relations in the NHS may be changing. It describes how changes in policy and professional discourses may have changed the nature of trust relations in the UK NHS and examines how changes in the organization and delivery of healthcare as well as broader social changes may have affected these relationships. A theoretical framework is presented for understanding the nature of trust relations between patients and healthcare professionals, between clinicians, and between healthcare professionals and managers. It concludes by a discussion of some of the methodological challenges involved with exploring the explanatory power of this framework empirically.

Chapter 3 examines the role of trust in relationships between patients and healthcare professionals, drawing on the published literature and the findings of the authors' research study which seeks to explore how trust relations differ for patients with an acute condition from those with a long-term health problem. It also explores the relationship between 'felt' and 'enacted' trust and how the concept of 'informed trust' and 'conditional trust' manifest themselves in people's accounts.

As the delivery of healthcare becomes more reliant on teamworking between health professionals, trust may be increasingly important to their relationships but inter-professional trust relations have been neglected in empirical research. Chapter 4 addresses the role of trust in relationships between different clinicians, what is considered high and low trust behaviour and what affects levels of trust between professionals. Findings from the research study examine the similarities and differences in how trust operates between healthcare professionals in an acute setting compared to those in primary care.

Chapter 5 explores the role of trust in relationships between managers, clinicians and patients. The increase in mechanisms to enhance accountability and the use of performance management and financial incentives for meeting central targets have generated new dependencies between clinicians and managers in which trust may play an important role. The chapter presents findings on trust in managerial–clinical relationships and to a lesser extent between managers and patients.

With the growth of patient choice in determining selection of provider, institutional trust is increasingly salient for healthcare organizations. Public trust in the NHS as an institution is similarly relevant to the sustainability of a tax-financed and publicly provided healthcare system. Chapter 6 examines the nature of public trust in healthcare institutions (both organizations and healthcare systems). It considers what builds and sustains institutional trust, how interpersonal trust may be reflected in institutional trust, and how trust in the NHS as a system links to the individual patient experience.

Chapter 6, the final chapter, also summarizes the conclusions from the different elements of the book and identifies the policy implications that flow from the empirical evidence and the evaluation of the theoretical framework. It also sets out a new agenda for research into trust relations in healthcare in the light of the analysis presented in this book.

NOTES

1 The correlations between the questions on levels of trust and those on confidence were consistently positive and strong, for example

- general practitioners .60
- hospital specialists .48
- health service managers .69
- nurses .60

This may suggest that trust and confidence are closely related and, as Rose-Ackerman (2001) suggests, while there may be a logical distinction between trust (intentional) and confidence (competence) it might not prevent trust implying confidence or at least embracing it.

2

TRUST IN THE NHS:
THEORETICAL PERSPECTIVES

INTRODUCTION

In the UK NHS trust has traditionally played an important part in the relationships between patients, clinicians and the government. The post-war consensus was underpinned by trust in professionalism (Newman 1998) with the state and patients tending to trust the norms of professional self-regulation and state licensing procedures to ensure that health professionals and healthcare institutions operated in the best interests of patients and citizens. However, in recent years it is claimed that, for a number of reasons, public trust in health institutions and in healthcare practitioners is in decline (Mechanic 2004). This chapter seeks to address how and why trust relations in the NHS may be changing, assessing the implications of various policy initiatives for trust relations in healthcare and presents a theoretical framework for exploring them in empirical research. Current discourses regarding a decline in trust are considered in light of ongoing debates as to whether medical power is in decline and the chapter concludes with a discussion of some of the methodological implications of exploring empirically the explanatory power of the concepts in the theoretical framework.

THE CONTEXT – THE 'NEW NHS'

Public and patient trust in healthcare in the UK appears to be shaped by a variety of factors. From a macro perspective, any changes in levels of public trust in healthcare institutions appear to derive partly from top-down policy initiatives that have altered the way in which health services are organized and partly from broader social and cultural processes which are claimed to have produced a decline in deference to authority and trust in experts and institutions, increasing reliance on personal judgements of risk, and which may be linked to an overall decline in social trust due to the breakdown of communities, social networks and cohesion. Consumerist forces it is proposed have produced a shift in the balance of power within which trust relations are formed, changing public and professional vulnerabilities and the requirement for trust in their relationships (Newman 1998). Institutional trust has also been affected by negative media coverage of scandals over medical competence in the 1990s. The change in public attitudes towards professionals and the emergence of more informed and potentially demanding patients that may have occurred as a result of these broader cultural processes provide a context for government policy which has positioned itself as seeking to make the NHS both more responsive to patients' needs, more efficient and more accountable for the quality of care provided. Any change in interpersonal and institutional trust relations can be understood as the natural outcome of these wider changes in both government policy and social attitudes.

In a later section we present a framework that seeks to demonstrate how changes in government policy regarding how to effectively govern the NHS may have resulted in changes in trust in the health system. A number of key policy initiatives are examined which we argue have changed the context for trust relations within the NHS including the introduction of clinical governance and the resulting use of performance management to scrutinize, change, and increase the accountability of clinical activity, and increasing patient choice and involvement in decision-making regarding their care. The implications of possible changes in the structure and nature of trust relations for the medical professions are considered in the light of current sociological debates regarding professionalism in medicine.

THE EFFECTS OF DIFFERENT GOVERNANCE MODELS ON TRUST IN HEALTHCARE

Table 2.1 sets out a theoretical framework that seeks to explain how changes in public trust in the health system may have been generated by different modes of governance of healthcare.

The framework is based on the proposition that changes in trust relations reflect changes to the distribution of power, modes of governance[1] and accountability within the health service. Changes to systems of governance invariably affect the distribution of power between various actors; they determine the systems and structures through which accountability is supposed to operate, and they reflect different levels of trust. For example, low levels of trust are implicit within certain approaches to governance such as new public management with its emphasis on greater regulation and surveillance and less discretion in work tasks (Fox 1974). The framework suggests that changes in trust are driven by the dialectical relationship between trust, power, governance and accountability, so that each affects the other in a continuing iterative process. Power is fundamental to trust relations wherein one party is dependent on the other; without such vulnerability trust would not be necessary. Fox (1974) argues that those holding power can show differing levels of trust and distrust by the extent to which they impose rules and regulations and limit the discretion of those dependent on them. Power is also fundamental to the understanding of accountability and governance; in a democracy public accountability is meaningless if the public does not have the power either directly or through its intermediaries to scrutinize the actions and performance of state agencies and to be able to seek redress. Trust has an inverse relationship with demands for explicit accountability; high trust relations result in limited demands for evidence of accountability and low trust relations produce increased demands for explicit evidence of the same. Thus, any changes to governance mechanisms that seek to increase accountability will produce shifts in the extent and distribution of power and trust in relations between patients, healthcare professionals and the state.

Within this conceptual framework the conditions in the post-war NHS exemplify the bureaucratic and professional models of governance outlined in Table 2.1 with high levels of trust between all three actors. However in the 1970s and 1980s it is claimed that this consensus began to disintegrate due to a combination of factors: changes in public attitudes and expectations of health professionals; the erosion of the 'mythical public service ethos' due to the promotion of entrepreneurial cultures in the public sector; and political and media portrayals of professional activity as paternalistic and flawed. In the 1990s trust in healthcare professionals is believed to have further declined due to intense media scrutiny about scandals over medical competence, such as the Inquiry into paediatric cardiac surgery in Bristol, the conviction of the GP Harold Shipman, and the removal of organs from children at Alder Hey Hospital. Lower levels

Table 2.1 Governance models and their impact on public trust in the UK NHS

Model	Organisational structure	Form of governance	Trust	Power	Accountability mechanisms	Lay power to hold health agencies to account
Bureaucratic	Integrated hierarchy	Command and control	High – trust in public service ethos and professionalism	Centralized – under political control	Political – reliant on ministerial accountability, line management and trust in public service ethos	Indirect – through periodic voting in elections
Professional	Self-regulating groups of relatively autonomous professionals	Network relations based on trust and mutual reciprocity	High – trust in professional expertise and norms	Dispersed – professional control	Professional – reliant on trust in professional integrity, guaranteed through licensing and disciplinary procedures	Generally passive recipients of care – complaints system only avenue to hold professionals to account
Market	Self-governing units in competition with each other	Exchange relations	Low in trust of professional and public service norms	Dispersed – consumer control	Economic – reliant on market forces to ensure 'responsiveness' – low in trust	Direct consumer action – through the exercise of choice and exit

New public management	Devolved operational units under centralized strategic control	'Tight–loose' relations with central steering at a distance	Low in trust – performance to be explicitly accounted for	Centralized – managerial control	Managerial – reliant on performance management against centrally determined targets – low in trust	Indirect – public views used to enhance organizational credibility and for organizational learning, but mediated by professionals
Stakeholder	Local agencies led by front-line providers with devolved autonomy but under central strategic control	Partnership working involving network relations based on trust and mutual reciprocity	High – trust in partner's respect of reciprocal rights and duties	Dispersed – stakeholder control	Multiple accountabilities – reliant on consultation, effective reporting and active involvement of stakeholders	Direct – active citizens are involved in service planning – public is a key constituency that agencies need to consult and be accountable to

Source: Rowe and Calnan 2006.

of trust may also be linked with how the NHS is run and financed and the pressure on NHS budgets due to increased demand by an ageing population, the rising costs of technology, and increases in public sector pay (Taylor-Gooby and Hastie 2003). Political concerns about a loss of public trust in professionalism, as a guarantor of high standards of conduct and competence, has prompted a debate about the accountability of clinicians, challenged the legitimacy of their power as enshrined in their right to clinical autonomy and high levels of discretion in their work, and has prompted a search for new mechanisms of governance to hold institutions and professionals accountable (Maynard and Bloor 2003).

The major thrust of policy in the 1990s was to use first market modes of governance with the creation of self-governing trusts and fundholding in general practice to introduce some contestability into the market, and then increasingly new public management mechanisms in an attempt to make the NHS more responsive and efficient. In the early years of the Labour administration in the 1990s, the government appeared to favour stakeholder approaches to governance as exemplified by Health Action Zones and Primary Care Groups which were underpinned by communitarian values that emphasized inclusion, participation and partnership working which could build trust between agencies and between the public and state institutions (Giddens 1990). Accountability and trust are achieved in this model through an ongoing dialogue between an organization and its stakeholders in which stakeholders can actively contribute to decision-making and ensure their interests are considered. However, political concerns to be able to report improvement in performance have tended to eclipse such initiatives with the government increasingly using performance management approaches to achieving accountability for both financial and clinical performance by introducing more formalized and explicit mechanisms of governance: specifications, standards, inspection, audit and monitoring, all under the direction of central government. In a final policy turn the Labour government have returned to the use of market mechanisms of governance, promoting provider competition to try to secure improvements in providers' effectiveness and productivity.

Figure 2.1 illustrates how the type of governance approach can produce different levels of trust and suggests that neither new public management techniques nor market mechanisms will be effective in increasing public trust in the health service. It raises the question whether complex systems of accountability and control undermine trust, displacing it with various criteria of performance and indicators

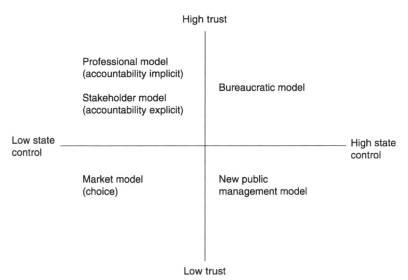

Figure 2.1 The distribution of trust and state control in various models of governance

Source: Rowe and Calnan (2006).

for review and accounting, or whether this new form of regulation encourages new strategies for building trust, and challenges the powerful expert/lay divide in healthcare and the concept of professionalism itself. In the next section we examine in more detail how performance management in the clinical domain and the expansion of patient choice of provider have affected trust relations within the NHS.

TRUST, CLINICAL GOVERNANCE AND PERFORMANCE MANAGEMENT

The introduction of 'clinical governance' in 1997 was a radical policy which arguably had the potential to create profound change in the relationships between clinicians and managers in the UK, in the process adjusting the political settlement agreed between the government and the medical professionals in 1948. When the NHS was established Nye Bevan granted physicians a monopoly of expertise to secure their support for a national health service, including the right to control entry to practice and autonomy over their clinical work in exchange for guaranteeing adequate standards of performance and integrating rationing decisions into clinical management (Klein 1996). Professional autonomy ensured that fully qualified physicians should not just have control over diagnosis and treatment for individual patients but should have control over the nature and volume of medical tasks and control over evaluation of care (Schulz and Harrison 1986). Under this professional model of accountability professionals operated within a network system of governance with authority relationships based not on hierarchy and line management but professional status, coordinative competence and resource control. Accountability was sustained through associational relations that relied on shared values and norms and an internal adherence to agreed ethical codes of conduct. Trust was central to this system. To be effective it required patients and politicians to have high levels of trust in the expertise of doctors and the effectiveness of professional self-regulation as a mechanism for ensuring high standards of care. For, in effect, self-regulation protected physicians from accounting to anyone other than their professional colleagues for their clinical activity and performance or use of resources, essentially rendering them invisible to public scrutiny (Evetts 1999).

The post-war consensus in the UK NHS in which trust in professionalism underpinned the relationships between the public, health professions and the State (Newman 1998) is believed to have been undermined by the growth of consumerism, an erosion of the public service ethos due to the promotion of entrepreneurial values in the public sector (Brereton and Temple 1999), and by political and media portrayals of professional activity as paternalistic. In the 1990s the public's trust in the ability of the medical profession's system of self-regulation to guarantee an appropriate quality of care appeared to decline. Notwithstanding the limited empirical evidence of an actual as opposed to a claimed decline, the apparent loss in public trust has been attributed to a number of factors, not least a series of high-profile clinical failures in the 1990s. The changing attitude of the public towards professionals and professional regulatory bodies is reflected in a more critical view of bodies such as the General Medical Council (GMC) which have appeared 'too much of a cosy club protective of medical interests' (Klein 1998: 154) rather than a vehicle that can ensure that professionals operate in the public interest. Old systems of self-regulation were seen as flawed in their ability to identify poorly performing healthcare professionals, particularly given the tendency for the profession to close ranks against 'whistle-blowers' (Hunt 1995; Taylor 1998). There is evidence to suggest that the public increasingly see the doctors' regulatory body, the GMC, as self-interested even though public trust in doctors remains high (Allsop 2006). For example, Allsop (2006) shows that over the last decade complaints to the NHS and the GMC and claims for negligence show an increasing trend and a betrayal of trust is a common reason given for making a complaint.

As traditional mechanisms to ensure professional accountability have lost public confidence, the government was able to use this opportunity to revise its settlement with the medical professions, introducing clinical governance as a mechanism to achieve clinical accountability for the quality of care provided and using performance management to influence how services are organized and delivered. This has been described as the 'hard' form or narrative of the new public management which aims to control public service professions through the introduction of an 'accounting logic' and an emphasis on audit, performance measurement and management, and performance related pay. More recently it has been suggested that a second narrative has become popular which is a softer or subtler version of the new public management and is associated with the human relations school of private sector management (Ferlie and Geraghty 2007). The emphasis here is on user orientation, quality improvement and organizational and individual development and learning. It still aims to move control and decision-making away from professionals although with the idea to absorb professionals into management systems.

Clinical governance was introduced as a framework within which local NHS organizations could work to improve and assure the quality of clinical services for patients and to minimize the risks of the negative consequences of healthcare outcomes. All NHS organizations are now required to develop processes for continuously monitoring and improving the quality of healthcare and to develop systems of accountability for the quality of care that they provide. While quality assurance and quality improvement are the two core strands to clinical governance, its objective was to increase clinical accountability. Hitherto, the medical profession had resisted political and managerial definitions of and approaches to quality assurance arguing that they cannot be applied to the 'uncertainties and ambiguities of clinical practice' (Degeling et al. 1998: 3). The professional approach to quality assurance had been through medical audit which has been voluntary, local and the preserve of medical specialists (Pollitt 1993). Clinical audit was seen as a learning process to facilitate professional development, a heuristic tool to improve practice. With the introduction of clinical governance, quality assurance and quality improvement processes are no longer closed activities entrusted to professionals. Instead government-led definitions of quality, in the form of guidance from the National Institute of Health and Clinical Excellence (NICE) and National Service Frameworks issued by the Department of Health, have been married to managerial procedures to secure clinical accountability. The quality of clinical work is benchmarked against nationally determined standards and subject to external scrutiny through the publication of performance data (NHSE 1999) with quality control procedures monitored by an external agency, currently the Healthcare Commission. These differences in quality improvement in the NHS before and after clinical governance are summarized in Table 2.2.

Clinical governance represents a substantial challenge to the authority of the medical profession as in theory it requires clinicians to account for what care is provided, the standards of that care, and how that care is organized and delivered. Moreover, the criteria against which clinical performance is measured are no longer exclusively and privately determined by clinicians and their professional bodies. Central government has been able to specify what services are to be provided and to what standard (Department of Health 2002) and these standards are increasingly being incorporated into commissioning agreements with hospitals and GPs so that in future their remuneration may depend on compliance with a list of highly specific quality indicators. Inspections by the Healthcare Commission, which include a review of clinical performance and the extent of

Table 2.2   Quality improvement pre- and post-clinical governance

Pre-clinical governance	*Post-clinical governance*
Voluntary	Mandatory
Closed professional activity	Open to external scrutiny
Locally determined standards set by professionals	Nationally determined standards set by government-led professional bodies
Professional accountability processes	Managerial accountability processes
High trust	Low trust

Source: Rowe and Calnan (2006).

compliance with NICE guidance, have increased surveillance of physicians' activity and require them to provide evidence of continuous quality improvement work. However, the way in which clinical governance has been implemented, using a softer form of public management, suggests that the radical potential for clinical governance has been sacrificed to achieve clinical engagement with the policy.

Increasing managerial monitoring of clinical activity linked to the clinical governance initiative has obvious consequences for trust relationships between providers and managers (Davies 1999) and potentially between local healthcare delivery organizations and the centre. Harrison and Smith (2004) argue that the new policy framework of clinical governance has sought to achieve a shift in focus from trust relationships between people to confidence in abstract systems, such as rules and regulations. The more behaviour is constrained by such systems so uncertainty is reduced and visibility is increased (Giddens 1990), the less we need to rely on trust (Smith 2001). Davies and Mannion (2000) have proposed that this possible shift from trusting in intrinsic professional motivation for the delivery of high-quality services to trust in performance management systems, which seek to provide data on the quality of healthcare, may have negative effects on the cultural intangibles that promote quality care, as well as the cost of information and accountability systems. The perverse incentives that may be generated by performance management systems, in that a system that 'does not trust people begets people that cannot be trusted' (Davies and Lampel 1998: 159), highlights the risk of gaming behaviour in such an approach.

It is also far from certain that credible external performance measurements build up confidence in organizations, requiring less trust in them. As Sheaff et al. (2004) noted in their scoping exercise for the Service Development Organization (SDO), there has been limited empirical research evaluating the impact of external performance measures, particularly from the perspective of service users. Those studies that have explored this problem have reported quite negative findings. Mannion and Goddard's (2003) evaluation of the impact of the Clinical Resources and Audit group (CRAG) clinical outcome indicators in Scotland reported limited use of such data by patients and GPs and also within hospital trusts. Similarly, studies of the use of US report cards have found on the whole that published performance data rarely stimulate quality improvement (Marshall et al. 2000) and the public distrusts and fails to make use of it (Schneider and Lieberman 2001). As Power (1997: 145) argues, the growth of performance measurement and audit may merely result in 'certificates of comfort' offering reassurance that performance is being measured without resulting in change. Thus, 'giving an account is seen to be a way of avoiding an account' (Day and Klein 1987: 171). It has also been suggested that the use of managers' resources in monitoring and surveillance may have reduced organizational effectiveness as they have fewer resources with which to accomplish fundamental work objectives (McAllister 1995). Where trust is low the reliability of information published may be questioned and any uncertainty in the data and what it means may do little to increase public confidence in healthcare institutions. Obtaining a performance measure that is credible to clinicians, commissioners and service users, and that enhances confidence in healthcare organizations, is particularly pertinent in the context of patient choice (Department of Health 2004a) to which we now turn.

TRUST AND PATIENT CHOICE

The introduction of patient choice illustrates how changes in the way services are commissioned and delivered can affect trust relations between patients, clinicians and managers. Patient choice has moved to the centre of the UK government's programme of health system reform as is well illustrated in the recent Green Papers on public health (2004) and adult social care (Department of Health 2005). However, choice has long been a problematic concept and the focus of debates as to whether an effective market for healthcare as a commodity can be established given the existence of externalities, uncertainty and information deficits regarding the cost, quantity and quality of care, and difficulties in entering and exiting the market (Calnan et al. 1993). Irrespective of whether the government's choice initiative is a pragmatic attempt to make health services more responsive or is tied to 'New Labour' values of applying 'what works' in the private sector to 'modernize' public services, it raises new issues in relation to trust. A core part of this programme is 'choose and book', which aims to give patients more choice on how, when and where they receive treatment for elective care. From the summer of 2004 all patients waiting more than six months were to be offered an alternative hospital for faster treatment and from December 2005 all patients in England are supposed to be offered four or five places for elective care. This was extended in April 2008 to patients being able to choose any provider who meets Health

Commission standards and can provide care at the nationally agreed price. The rationale for greater patient choice is to increase the responsiveness of the NHS to service users. In theory, rather than passively trusting GPs' recommendations regarding referral for specialist treatment, patients will be able to participate in decisions about where to go for treatment and when.

However, instead of negating the need for trust, the individualization of commissioning through 'choose and book' makes both institutional trust and trust in specific healthcare practitioners even more salient. As Mannion and Smith (1996) reported in their study of the community care market, choice and contracts do not obviate the need for trust, particularly when dealing with complex products such as health and social care which are characterized by informational difficulties and uncertainties and a marketplace in which purchasers are risk averse. Where choice is a meaningful option, secondary care hospitals may find that their financial viability may depend on levels of patients' and GPs' trust in them as institutions. Patient choice will influence financial flows in the NHS as choice is being linked to 'payment by results' whereby payment of providers is linked to activity, with money flowing with the patient. As providers in the USA have experienced, sustaining trust may be something hospitals need to actively facilitate in order to encourage patient loyalty and ensure financial survival. A patient's trust in their individual GP will be all the more important, not just for the potential therapeutic benefits, but because they may rely on them to interpret performance data in making referral decisions. Data regarding the waiting times and clinical outcomes of different providers may need to be explained before patients are able to use such information to make a decision as to choice of referral. However, while some GPs may be willing to explain such data, others may rely on more traditional bases for recommending a provider such as their personal knowledge of the doctors leading the service. Mannion and Smith (1996) found that purchasers' choice of residential home was influenced by their reputation for trustworthiness, because of the lack of information on quality, and that their views on the reputation of providers were based on the informal networks among care managers rather than the results of formal inspections.

Choice also requires GPs to have increased trust in patients, that they are able to make an informed decision about where to go for a referral and in some cases that they will make the referral themselves (if they decide to book an appointment electronically after their GP consultation). In a feasibility study of GPs offering choice for routine adult surgical referrals, Taylor et al. (2004) found that there were significant delays in making the referral while patients considered their options. The same study showed that only 22 per cent of doctors in the study offered choice all or most of the time and that most patients still opted for their local hospital. In an evaluation of London patient choice, which involved patients waiting for elective surgery, one in three patients were critical of the amount and quality of information they had received (Ellins 2005). Of the third of patients who declined the offer of choice, many said that they had been given insufficient information to enable them to make an informed decision. Variations in such health literacy may exacerbate health inequalities over choice and to avoid this additional resources may be required in the form of patient care advisers to guide patients through the choice process. Research is needed to identify the extent to which patient trust in their local healthcare organizations and in the recommendations of their GP influences choice; such decisions could be an expression of trust as much as an expression of choice. Empirical research is also required to understand how institutional trust can be generated and sustained as the financial viability of secondary care providers may depend on their ability to develop trust-building activities with primary care providers and the communities they serve.

TRUST AND PATIENT PARTICIPATION IN DISEASE MANAGEMENT

While Labour's policy of involving patients in referral decisions regarding secondary care is relatively new, initiatives to involve patients in decision-making about managing their own condition, particularly those with chronic health problems, are well established. Trust relationships are particularly important in chronic disease management as trust is known to be important for adherence with medical advice in the chronically ill (Mosley-Williams et al. 2002; Lukoschek 2003) and it is considered a core component of effective therapeutic relationships (Dibben and Lena 2003). Successful management of many chronic diseases depends at least as much on changes that the patient can make as it does on specific medical interventions, and as a result requires a partnership between patient and health professional. Some studies have explored the evolving nature of trust relations between clinicians and patients with chronic disease, seeking to identify how trust is built and sustained in the

therapeutic alliance (Thorne and Robinson 1988, 1989). Their findings suggest that trust in clinicians varies according to the stage of
the disease and the point in its treatment. Trust appears to depend not
just on a provider's demonstration of care and concern for the patient
as an individual, it also requires clinicians to show confidence in a
patient's ability to manage their disease (Thorne and Robinson1989;
Kai and Crosland 2001; Henman et al. 2002). Being viewed as competent by a healthcare professional encouraged patients to feel more
confident in their ability to control and manage their illness and at
the same time increased patient trust in the provider.

These findings are highly pertinent to current UK policy which is
encouraging patient self-management as part of its programme to
reduce the burden of chronic disease (Department of Health 2004a)
and the costs to the health service (Taylor and Bury 2007). In order
to stimulate activity in this area, chronic disease management has
been identified as key to improving the quality and performance of
general practice. This is reflected in the new General Medical
Services (GMS) contract which includes specific payments for practices to proactively manage patients with chronic disease through its
new quality framework (Department of Health 2003). This forms
part of the policy implemented in the UK in 2004 when general
practitioners were given substantial financial incentives to meet a
range of clinical and organizational targets known as the 'Quality
and Outcomes Framework' (QOF) (Roland 2004). The Government's chronic disease management programme has important
implications for trust relations: requiring providers to increase their
trust in patients' ability for self-care; encouraging more integrated
approaches to service delivery between providers involved in disease
and case management; and involving managers from primary care
organizations who are responsible for assessing and rewarding practices' standards of activity in this area (Department of Health 2002).
The success of this policy is of course dependent on a patient's
willingness and ability to participate in decision-making, which in
turn reflects wider changes in public attitudes and expectations of
health professionals.

The policy initiatives outlined above, we would argue, have produced a new context for trust relations within the NHS, shifting
the interdependence and distribution of power between patients,
clinicians and managers and changing their vulnerability to each
other and to healthcare institutions.

PROFESSIONALISM, CLAIMS MAKING AND TRUST

The debate about the decline or not in trust in healthcare and modern medicine and potential changes in trust relations should not be divorced from the broader discussion in the sociology of professionalism which has focused on the extent to which medical power and authority is in decline or that medicine has, in the face of recent challenges, managed to retain its overall dominance. Those advocating that medical power is on the wane highlight the threats generated through the impact of the processes of proletarianization, deprofessionalization, corporatization and bureaucratization. For example, Coburn et al. (1997) argued that manageralism has undermined the profession as whole through the state co-option of medical organizations and élites. They argue that medical institutions are being used by external forces, such as the State, to constrain their own members and to implement policies over which they have no control. Alternative and contrasting sociological accounts of the professionalizing strategies of medicine have argued how, at least at the élite or macro level, it is able to respond to or anticipate possible challenges or changes, and sometimes use the opportunities to maintain or even enhance its autonomy and control. For example, Friedson (1994; 2001) puts forward a theory of professional re-stratification which suggests increasing divisions between the rank and file of doctor practitioners and the 'knowledge' (research) and administrative medical élites. Friedson (1994; 2001) argues that while the power base may have shifted within the profession towards these élite groups, the profession itself was still dominant. For example, the élite practitioners and medical researchers play a central role in developing the clinical protocols and guidelines being used by the rank and file practitioners, and the increasing number of medical doctors taking on managerial roles suggests that doctors may be taking back the professions' monitoring and regulatory roles.

The analysis of the policy discourses presented previously suggests that medicine has been coerced into changes in the structure and nature of trust relations. For example, as Allsop shows (2006), the UK government in the late 1990s stated that there was a clear need for the current structure of professional self-regulation to change (Department of Health 1998: 3.44) 'Recent events have dented public confidence in the quality of clinical care provided by the NHS. The challenge for the profession is to demonstrate that professional self-regulation can continue to enjoy public confidence.'

A similar theme runs through the current professional 'discourse' on trust in that the so-called decline in public trust brought about by scandals such as Shipman is a 'problem' for medicine and has led to the introduction of tighter mechanisms for regulation and account-ability. Yet, it is difficult to know how far these changes were forced on the profession or whether it, or certain sections of it, may have colluded with the state as it enhanced their project of modernizing medicine and public services (Smith 1992).

Certainly, there have been changes in the organization and remit of the General Medical Council (Allsop 2006) which appears to have been a response to the media reporting of the failings of a small number of clinicians (Flynn 2002). More recently in changes in regulatory policy from the Chief Medical Officer (Department of Health 2006), the emphasis was placed on proposals for revalidation with changes to existing systems of licensure and certification of doctors which would involve regular assessments of their skills, practice and conduct against clearly defined standards. In addition, the 'modern medical professions' representatives appear to be advocating value-based as opposed to representative leadership associating themselves with the philosophy of the 'new professionalism', and central to this is a call to the public for a partnership based on mutual trust. The old concordat between the profession, the State and the public founded on self-regulation and paternalism would be replaced with a new one based on patient autonomy and patients' rights, and greater accountability on the part of doctors and partnership. Thus, it appears to be no coinci-dence that the most recent government proposals on regulation are entitled 'Trust, Assurance and Safety' (Department of Health 2007). This approach might be seen as another example of a professional-izing strategy in that it is a way of heading off any further threats to autonomy by the State or through marketization by emphasizing the need for patients to trust doctors to self-regulate and to work together with them. In the past professionalism and trust were pre-sumed to be intrinsic to doctors' values and the doctor–patient rela-tionship, whereas now professional bodies or their representatives feel the need to make them explicit. Clearly, they also saw a need for professionalism as an occupational value in its own right to be restated and made explicit.

This development resonates with sociological arguments which suggest that there is an emergence or re-emergence of trust in socio-logical theories of occupational development and control as well as an appeal to the discourse of professionalism. Previous critical analysis of professionalism depicted occupations as driven primarily by self-interest and the need for power, status and material wealth rather than altruism. Trust was used as a means for duping or coercing the public into believing in the superior product of scientific medicine and thus enhancing the professionalizing project. More recent theories have reconnected trust and professionalism through the renewed interest in risk and the challenges posed by a possible decline in public trust. For example, as Evetts (2006) suggests, the current appeal to professionalism for occupations has markedly different implications from the more traditional type of occupational control which medicine exemplified over 50 years ago. The appeal to professionalism most often includes the substitution of organizational for professional values, accountability replacing trust and autonomy being constrained and controlled. 'Professionalism and trust become important once again because trust is perceived to be in serious decline' (Evetts 2006: 525).

Other sociological accounts of the link between trust and professionalism have shown how the medical profession have used the development of external regulation such as guidelines to reinforce their professional position. They suggest that the development of these new tools of bureaucratic regulation which are signifiers of quality are actively used by doctors to build trustful relations with colleagues. They are used as 'public proofs' of quality of their services under conditions of tighter control and regulation. They are also taken up by patients and perceived as prerequisites for self-determined decisions and trustworthy relations. The traditional 'embodied' professionalism is transformed into a 'disembodied' professionalism founded on information. Thus, Kuhlmann (2006) argues that new patterns of building trust are emerging rather than in decline. On this premise, exhortations by senior leaders within the medical profession for their colleagues to engage with and lead implementation of 'clinical governance' may be interpreted as a further way of clinicians seeking to protect their power base. Clinicians may be more explicitly accountable for the quality of care they provide but they continue to define what quality is, how it is to be measured and how the results can be interpreted. Thus, professional regulation may have become a fragmented mixture of self and external controls.

The sociology of professionalism also embraces the position and perspective of the patient, client or layperson and, as previous discussions have suggested, there have been developments which may influence trust relations with both providers and managers. One of these developments involved the emergence of the so-called lay 'expert'. Empirical research (Calnan 1987) has shown for some time that in some contexts and clinical settings (typically chronic illness and disability) patients or their representatives become knowledgeable when they recognize that medicine has little to offer and they search for other sources of knowledge and help. However, lay knowledge as a concept became more generally accepted when sociologists and anthropologists attempted to shift accounts of illness and health-related behaviour away from positivistic and individualistic explanations to those which have put an emphasis on the pluralistic and interpretative nature of the social world. There was, however, as Prior et al. (2003) point out, an apparent shift over this period in the way the category of lay knowledge was conceptualized or formulated. Peoples' beliefs about cause shifted or evolved into the sturdier notion of lay knowledge, and lay concepts of aetiology and disease causation turned into a focus on lay epidemiology and the emergence of the notion of the 'lay' expert. 'A concern with belief had been transposed into a concern with knowledge and that lay people had metamorphosed into multi-skilled and knowledgeable individuals' (Prior 2003: 45).

Other commentators also identified the emergence of the lay expert but depicted it in terms of or juxtaposed it against the decline in trust in professional scientific medicine. This is believed to reflect changes in public attitudes, values and expectations of healthcare practitioners (Sztompka 1999; Salter 2000) and technology brought about, at least in part, by wider social and cultural changes. These might include the decline in deference to authority and trust in experts and institutions, and increasing reliance on personal judgements of risk (Giddens 1990; Beck 1992; O'Neill 2002), where active forms of trust and radical forms of doubt have become a pervasive feature of modern critical reasoning (Williams and Calnan 1996) or the overall decline in social trust due to breakdown in communication, social networks and cohesion (Putnam 2000). A related theme is the belief that the structure of the doctor–patient relationship has changed and the most popular form now is a 'shared' rather than 'paternalistic' relationship, where the patient is more active and involved in decision-making (Stewart and Roter 1989; Mead and Bower, 2000). This has been brought about by the increasing accessibility of medical knowledge through the mass media and the Internet (Hardey 1999) which has led to a challenge to the traditional, hierarchical professional lay relationship due to the closing of the gap in knowledge between the professional expert and the lay person.

The emergence of the lay expert, however, may reflect a change rather than a decline in trust relations as theorists and those involved in empirical research appear to suggest that the public hold a contradictory or ambivalent position about scientific medicine. For example, as Lupton (1994) argues, Western societies in the late twentieth century are characterized by people's increasing disillusionment with scientific medicine and yet, paradoxically, there is also an increasing dependence on biomedicine to provide the answers to social as well as medical problems. Certainly, there seems to be a widespread suspicion of prescribed medicines (Horne et al. 1999) which stems from the perception that they are chemicals manufactured by large multinational industries. In this respect pharmaceuticals are often contrasted with complementary and alternative treatments which are perceived to be less harmful and (more appropriately) because they are 'natural'. This may account for the growing popularity of 'complementary' therapies, although this may also be due to its perceived benefits for chronic conditions where discrete pathology is elusive and complementary and alternative medicine (CAM) treatments are perceived to be safer. On the other hand, it is equally clear that the 'lay' public still continue to look to medicine for a solution to their ills. High-technology medicine, although not devoid of criticism tends to be greeted with a considerable degree of reverence and respect by the lay public (Williams and Calnan 1996). Even the growth of complementary therapy does not imply a wholesale rejection of orthodox medicine and dual usage remains very much the norm (Sharma 1995).

   In the following section we outline a theoretical framework which seeks to identify the different forms of trust relations that may be emerging in the context of a 'modernized' NHS based on current policy, professional and sociological discourses.

THEORETICAL FRAMEWORK FOR TRUST RELATIONS IN THE 'NEW NHS'

The following framework is based on the proposition that changes in the organizational structure of healthcare, the culture of healthcare delivery and specific policy initiatives have changed the experiences of healthcare for individual patients and affected trust relations between patients, providers and managers. These changes have in part been initiated by healthcare professionals, in part by the government and in part by patients, some of whom wish to be equal partners in treatment decisions. It is not proposed that these changes have cumulatively achieved a shift from trust in people to confidence in abstract systems. The provision of healthcare is still characterized by uncertainty and risk and there is evidence that not only are patients sceptical of institutional confidence-building mechanisms such as performance ratings, but that interactions between managers and clinicians continue to rely on informal relations and unwritten rules rather than performance management (Goddard and Mannion 1998). Rather, current policy and professional discourses suggest that new forms of trust relations are emerging in this new context of healthcare delivery, reflecting a change in motivations for trust from affect-based to cognition-based trust as patients, clinicians and managers become more active partners in trust relations.

For patients in the new NHS, embodied trust (Green 2004), arising out of an enduring relationship with the 'family doctor', may be less relevant now due to new points of access to healthcare such as walk-in centres, and as patients increasingly see any doctor and other clinicians such as the nurse practitioner in their practice rather than waiting to see their 'named' GP. For some patients, as their care may be provided by an increasing range of healthcare professionals, professional and educational credentials and status may no longer be sufficient guarantees that an individual clinician will provide the standard and type of care they want. It is possible that they may trust nurses or therapists to be competent in certain aspects of their care but for other aspects they insist on seeing a doctor. Rather than passively accepting the advice of their GP on how to manage their condition, they may turn to the Internet as an alternative source of information. It is proposed that provision of information and greater patient involvement in their care, through the attempted shift towards shared decision-making in doctor–patient relationships, has produced greater interdependence between patient and clinician making informed trust more relevant to the patient experience. However, this shift towards informed conditional trust is likely to vary according to the nature of the patient's illness as well as their willingness and ability to adopt this more 'active' stance and whether they have access to resources (finance, time, energy) to do this (Lupton 1996). It may be that the same patient may show relatively blind trust in some contexts and more informed trust in others, depending on their needs and circumstances. Conditional trust may be more prevalent in certain illness contexts; in Mechanic and Meyer's study (2000) patients with acute illnesses such as breast cancer were more likely to describe their trust relations as being unconditional than those with Lyme disease who had experienced difficulties in obtaining a diagnosis. Trust relations are also dynamic and may change during the pathway of care. Thorne and Robinson (1988) reported that patients went from having a naive, unconditional trust on diagnosis through to a more conditional, negotiated relationship as their treatment became more established. Levels of trust may also vary according to the complexity of care; where it is complex patients may develop close relations with their hospital doctors producing the 'thick trust' Putnam associates with relationships with friends and relatives than the thin trust associated with strangers.

For GPs and hospital doctors, their trust relations with other practitioners may have changed as the clinical and professional boundaries of nurses and other professions allied to medicine are shifting and other healthcare professionals become responsible for and have increasing discretion over the delivery of services, creating new relations in which trust has to be earned through collaboration rather than relying on traditional hierarchy. The extent of trust within clinical teams may be reflected by the quality of communication and knowledge sharing between practitioners and the extent to which non-medics have discretion in conducting their role and to exercise their judgement when treating patients. New trust relations may have also been created through the increased regulation of training and working hours for both senior and junior hospital doctors such as through the introduction of shift systems of working. This increased regulation, according to some researchers, has led hospital doctors in the NHS to have an increasing reliance and maybe trust in formal as opposed to experiential knowledge (Nettleton et al. 2008). The government's clinical governance policy has also created new interdependencies between clinicians and managers and new opportunities for trust in their relationships. For example, in general practice individual GPs have been required to develop closer relations with other practitioners, with practice nurses and with practice managers to ensure that they can provide performance data for primary care trust managers to reimburse them for meeting the Quality and Outcomes Framework targets in the new General Medical Services Contract. Similarly, primary care trust managers now rely on practices to achieve their centrally determined waiting time targets. The extent to which primary care trust managers and practices perceive their goals to be shared, in terms of meeting government-specified performance targets, may influence levels of trust in their relationship and how closely the work of practices is monitored. These new interdependencies may be stimulated by performance management but also create the opportunity for emerging forms of trust relationships as exemplified in Table 2.3. The framework suggests

Table 2.3 Conceptual framework for explaining trust relations in the new NHS

Relationship	Trustor		Trustee		Context	Type of trust
	Affect-based	Cognition-based	Reputation based on status	Reputation based on performance		
Traditional clinician–patient	X		X		Paternalistic medicine	Embodied trust
Traditional clinician–clinician		X	X		Autonomous self-regulation	Peer trust
Traditional clinician–manager	X		X		Professional autonomy/expertise	Status trust
New NHS clinician–patient	X	X	X	X	Expert patient	Informed trust
New NHS clinician–clinician	X	X		X	Shared care	Earned trust
New NHS clinician–manager		X		X	Clinical governance	Performance trust

Source: Rowe and Calnan (2006).

that trust relations in all three types of relationship in the 'new' modernized NHS might, in general, be particularly characterized by an emphasis on communication, providing information and the use of 'evidence' to support decisions in a reciprocal negotiated alliance.

METHODOLOGICAL IMPLICATIONS

The conceptual framework outlined above raises a number of methodological questions for future empirical research. If trust relations are typified by a more conditional trust, what indicators could be used to recognize it in healthcare organizations? What we might want to look for is how trust relations vary along a spectrum ranging from high unconditional trust to low trust or distrust, with conditional trust placed somewhere along this spectrum (see Figure 2.2).

Different levels of trust might be identified by examining a range of beliefs and attitudes, as exemplified in Table 2.4, that individual patients, clinicians and managers have about their relationships with other people and healthcare institutions that involve trust.

Existing instruments which have been developed to measure levels of trust may be able to identify levels that reflect more conditional trust relations, but there is a further methodological problem in that espoused levels of trust may vary from enacted trust levels. In order to allow for socially desirable responses, it may be more helpful for research to focus on enacted trust behaviour rather than espoused levels of trust. Following from this Table 2.5 outlines the possible behaviours which might be typified as manifesting high and low trust.

It was argued in the earlier part of the chapter that changes in national policy linked with changes in the position of professional medicine may have led to changes in trust relations in the NHS between patients practitioners and managers. The theoretical framework (see Table 2.3) typifies the new type of trust relations which may have emerged as a result of these changes but how can these changes be explored empirically? How might informed trust (see Table 2.3) be characterized from a patient's perspective and in what ways would it

Conditional trust

High, unconditional trust   Low trust/distrust

Figure 2.2   The trust continuum
Source: Rowe and Calnan (2006).

Table 2.4   Attitudes that reflect felt trust

High trust	Low trust
Belief that others will not harm us	Belief that others might harm us
Low levels of anxiety, suspicion and scepticism	High levels of anxiety, suspicion and scepticism
Limits to knowledge are acceptable	Limits to knowledge are not acceptable
Lack of control is acceptable	Lack of control is a problem
Draw comfort from relations	Anxious about relations

Source: Rowe and Calnan (2006).

differ from patients' perspectives on embodied trust? There are a number of possible dimensions (see Figure 2.3). One is clearly in the area of decision-making where there would be an increasingly active patient involved in decision-making who might expect doctors to trust their ability/competence to self-manage compared with the more passive and deferent role associated with paternalistic medicine. The second dimension involves the use of information. Informed trust might be associated with the use of information to calculate

Table 2.5   Behaviours that reflect trust

High trust behaviour	Low trust behaviour
Minimal checking	Constant monitoring
Informal, unwritten rules	Detailed and prescriptive regulations
Significant professional autonomy	Intense supervision and little delegation of authority
Willingness to take risks	Risk averse
Willingness to divulge information	Information is withheld
Passive, deferent role	Questioning, possibly sceptical role
Forgive errors and mistakes	Errors result in intense blame and complaints
Advice is accepted unquestioningly	Request for a second opinion or alternative source of treatment sought

Source: Rowe and Calnan (2006).

If trust is more *embodied* you would expect:
• Patients have a more passive, deferential role.
• Information is valued for the respect it shows rather than its content.
• Advice/recommendations are accepted unquestioningly.
• Trust relates to 'family'/'personal' experience of doctor.
• There is an association between the level of direct contact and level of trust.
• There is minimal checking or monitoring with managers and clinicians being given considerable autonomy in decision-making.
• Rules are unwritten, informal and processes are not prescriptive.
• There is an assumption that the other party is well intentioned towards you.
• A clinician's altruism is unquestioned.
• Willingness to take risks is based on the reputation of the organization or individual.

If trust is more *informed* you would expect the following beliefs and behaviours:
• Information is used to calculate whether trust is warranted.
• Careful monitoring, supervision and checking (possibly covert).
• Patients want to play a more equal role in decision-making.
• Patients expect doctors to trust their ability/competence to self-manage.
• Patients may be more questioning of treatment recommendations.
• They may express greater suspicion and scepticism about others' intentions.
• Willingness to take risks is based on careful weighing-up of the situation.

Figure 2.3   Embodied and informed trust: patients' beliefs and behaviour

whether trust is warranted whereas with 'embodied' trust information may have been valued for the respect it shows rather than its content. In this way, patients may display a rational response rather than an emotive response to information. Third, perspectives may differ on the willingness to take risks in that informed trust may involve the patient carefully weighing up the situation whereas embodied trust may involve the patient basing their judgement on the reputation of the organization or individual. Finally, embodied trust implies a clinician's altruism is unquestioned and the other party is well intentioned. This may be contrasted with informed trust where the patient may express greater suspicion and scepticism about others' intentions.

For clinicians, 'earned' trust (see Figure 2.4) might be characterized by: clinicians' authority and reputation being based on their proven skills and competence, and being up to date with medical technology; limits to clinical freedom with trust gained by following agreed team-based protocols; successful relations between clinicians based on mutual respect for their different competencies and knowledge; and communication skills and providing information. This stands in marked contrast to more traditional relations of 'peer trust' where an individual clinician's authority and reputation are based on their position in the medical hierarchy, personal networks and word-of-mouth recommendation. Hierarchical relations dominate as clinical

If trust is *'peer'* you might expect the following:
* Clinicians' authority and reputation are based on their position in the medical hierarchy, personal networks and word-of-mouth recommendation.
* Senior clinicians' views and decisions are unquestioned.
* Clinical freedom is unquestioned.
* Performance is self-regulated, individually assessed and not publicly reported.
* Complex patients are only seen by senior doctors.
* 'Successful' relations between clinicians are based on conforming to traditional roles.
* Trust is generally higher between clinicians of the same profession and specialism.

If trust is *'earned'* you might expect the following beliefs and behaviours:
* Clinicians' authority and reputation are based on their proven skills and competence, and being up-to-date with medical technology.
* Clinical freedom may be limited and trust gained by following agreed protocols and an ability to work well in a team.
* Careful performance monitoring against targets.
* Both complex and easy patients may be seen by junior clinicians on the basis that they are following agreed protocols.
* 'Successful' relations between clinicians are based on mutual respect for their different skills.
* Trust may be higher between clinicians who have experience of working together, irrespective of their profession or specialism.
* Communication skills and providing information are important in building trust.
* Junior clinicians may question the views of their seniors.

Figure 2.4   Peer and 'earned' trust: clinicians' beliefs and behaviours

freedom is unquestioned, as are senior clinicians' views and decisions, performance is self-regulated, and successful relations between clinicians are based on conforming to traditional roles. Trust may be generally higher between clinicians of the same profession and specialism.

With regard to changes in trust relations between managers and practitioners, we argue that this relationship has changed from one characterized by status to one characterized by 'performance' (see Table 2.3). The former might be depicted (see Figure 2.5) as a one-way relationship with clinicians having little need to trust managers whereas managers have to trust clinicians' intrinsic motivation to provide high standards of care. Clinicians' authority relates to their position and role within the organization and managers act as administrators, trusting strategic decisions as to how services are to be delivered and how resources are to be used to clinicians. There would be minimal monitoring of activity and the quality of care delivered and managers would not be involved in such assessments. In contrast, performance trust might involve a two-way relationship as clinicians need to work with managers to secure resources and to develop services, and managers have to work with clinicians to achieve

If trust is based on '*status*' you might expect the following beliefs and behaviours:
* Clinicians' authority relates to their position and role within the hospital/organization.
* Rules are unwritten and there is minimal monitoring of clinical activity.
* Trust is one way – clinicians have little need to trust managers whereas managers have to trust clinicians.
* In decision-making managers act as administrators, trusting strategic decisions regarding service development to clinicians.
* Managers are not involved in monitoring or checking clinical activity.

If trust is more based on '*performance*' you might expect the following:
* Clinicians' authority relates to their ability to meet targets as well as their position within the organization.
* Trust is likely to be higher in those clinicians who have some managerial role.
* A willingness to provide information on clinical activity and to engage with managerial agendas creates trust.
* In 'successful' clinician–manager relations trust is important because it reduces the need for checking and monitoring.
* Trust is two-way – clinicians need to work with managers to secure resources and to develop services.
* In decision-making managers work with clinicians to make strategic decisions about services.
* An evidence-based approach to clinical practice using guidelines and protocols encourages trust.

Figure 2.5   Status and performance trust: managers beliefs and behaviours

their performance goals and to meet government targets. Clinicians' authority would be related to their involvement in managerial activity including the provision of data on outcomes and their ability to meet targets, as well as their position within the organization and clinical skills. Trust would be important in successful clinician–manager relations as it reduces the need for monitoring and may produce greater job satisfaction, higher staff retention, and more efficient organizational performance.

Although survey instruments may be able to capture some of these dimensions of trust beliefs and behaviour, the conceptual complexity of trust and the lack of empirical research that has examined trust relations within the context of the UK NHS does suggest that qualitative methods need to be employed at least initially to inform our conceptual understanding of trust relations and trust behaviour (Strauss and Corbin 1998). In particular, research is needed to understand how macro-level processes, including provider–provider and provider–manager relations may constrain or enhance micro-level provider–patient trust relations, and how trust between individuals affects institutional trust. The relationship between trust beliefs and trust behaviour also needs to be examined, exploring how different expressions of trust might manifest themselves in behaviour.

This chapter has, through analysis of recent developments in health and health service policy, medical professional policy and sociological theories of professionalism, set out to show how and why trust relations in the NHS may be changing. A theoretical framework has been developed from this analysis which identifies what these new trust relations might look like. The final section has considered some of the methodological challenges to exploring trust relations and has specified how these concepts of trust relations may be explored empirically. The typical dimensions of what informed, earned, and performance trust might look like are described although little empirical research has been conducted to investigate the nature of trust relations within the UK health system. The following chapters present evidence from the authors' comparative case studies which assess the explanatory power of this framework and explore how far these concepts are salient and meaningful in trust relations between patients, practitioners and managers.

NOTES

1   Governance in this discussion is being used according to its definition: the action or manner of governing. In the new public management literature governance has been attributed a particular meaning: governance involves the state being responsible for contracting services from a wide range of agencies and stakeholders. As such it has been used to contrast with government whereby the state's role has been the direct provision of services.

3

TRUST BETWEEN PATIENTS AND CLINICIANS

In this chapter we examine the nature of patient trust in clinicians: nurses, doctors, healthcare assistants and therapists based in two very different organizational settings. Case study 1 comprised a GP surgery which was a training practice located in a working-class and deprived community in a large city and involved interviewing patients with type 2 diabetes about their trust relationships with the health professionals they came into contact within the practice. Case study 2 comprised two orthopaedic wards in a large acute hospital serving the same urban area and involved interviewing patients who had undergone elective surgery for a hip replacement. The different clinical conditions and organizational settings were purposively selected to explore whether and how trust relations are influenced by organizational and clinical context. We first describe the nature of trust relations in these two contrasting settings before examining specific aspects of patient trust in clinicians including the types of trust exhibited, how trust is built and lost, what constitutes high and low trust behaviour and the benefits and disadvantages of trust.

THE NATURE OF TRUST RELATIONS BETWEEN DIABETES PATIENTS AND CLINICIANS IN PRIMARY CARE

In the theoretical framework outlined in Chapter 2 we suggested that patients in the NHS today may exhibit less embodied trust which traditionally arose out of an enduring relationship with their 'family doctor'. With the end of personal lists for GPs and the expansion of primary care teams to include nurse practitioners, practice nurses and healthcare assistants, patients can see a range of professionals within the practice creating the opportunity for different points of access to healthcare. Easier access to medical information through the Internet and from disease-specific charities led us to propose that as diabetes patients can become expert in their own long-term condition then informed trust might be more relevant. Whether patients trust the clinicians who provide their diabetes care will depend on the extent and nature of information they provide and whether this meets patients' needs and does not conflict with their own knowledge of their condition. With a long-term condition like diabetes where patient self-management is important for symptom control, we also suggested that there could be greater interdependence between patients and clinicians, creating the need for more mutual trust rather than the traditional one-way trust of patients in doctors.

Our research in the urban practice described in the Appendix revealed that diabetes patients have trust relations with a variety of clinicians, both within the practice and beyond it in the local acute hospital (see Figure 3.1). Most patients talked at length about the need for mutual trust between individual clinicians and patients, especially between themselves and the lead diabetes nurse and between themselves and 'their GP'. Patients suggested that clinicians needed to trust them to follow the lifestyle changes they recommended and to take their medication appropriately while they needed to trust healthcare professionals to provide them with good clinical care.

> Male patient: Er yes, it is important to me that – that who I deal with trusts me.
> *When they say they trust you, what do they actually mean?*
> Well, that you're doing what they want you to do and you're doing it properly, as to medication.

Changes in social relations appear to be reflected in the doctor–patient relationship as clinicians recognized the need for greater mutual trust given their more respectful relationship with patients:

> Salaried GP: I certainly think there's increasing levels of trust that have been delegated to patients, and I think that's very good. And, following that, increasing levels of respect ... I think doctors haven't always had to trust patients ... doctors just did things to patients.

For some of these relationships trust was still embodied with two patients expressing blind trust in their 'family doctor', but for most

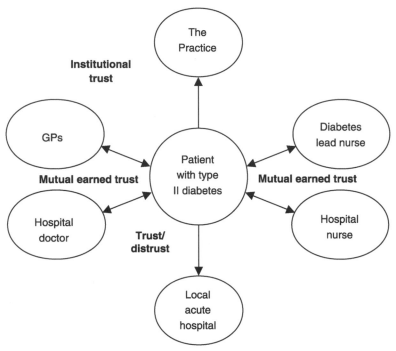

Figure 3.1 Trust relations between diabetic patients and clinicians in primary care

patients trust was conditional in that it had to be earned over time based on the care they received. Whether patients trusted the practice nurses or the GPs depended on their experience of care, including whether their treatment was successful, and to a lesser extent on the amount of time patients and clinicians had known each other. This does not depend on the type or amount of information they are given, as might be expected with 'informed trust', but on the nature of their relationship and their experience of care. Likewise, clinicians' trust in patients was earned by their ability to take medication as advised and make dietary changes as well as their behaviour in the surgery, whether they turned up for appointments, were polite and honest about their symptoms:

> Practice nurse: And also you need to be able to trust from a medication point of view; if you're asking them to take certain medications you have to trust that they're going to be able to take that appropriately and not have any mistakes or mishaps,

especially where diabetes is concerned . . . It's a bit of a two-way relationship really.

Only one male patient discounted trust as being important in his relationship with his doctor. He understood trust in terms of blind trust and considered that that was no longer appropriate:

> I don't think trust is of any importance any more . . . I think it's confidence in your doctor which I don't think that's the same necessarily as trust you know . . . I think it's very import-ant that you don't rely entirely on the doctor because we've got to have our own opinions about how to look after our own health.

When patients were questioned as to whether they trusted nurses differently to doctors, their trust varied according to the competen-cies of the healthcare professional. Thus, patients trusted doctors to diagnose and prescribe, while nurses were trusted to provide 'ongoing care'. Although the lead diabetes nurse was very skilled and managed the bulk of the diabetes caseload, several patients talked about requesting to see their GP as well to discuss the results of blood tests. Diabetes patients also referred to their relationship with hospital-based clinicians, suggesting that trust was again earned based on their experience of care but that it was sometimes harder to trust them because the team approach to care restricted relationship building:

> Diabetes patient 5: I do feel less comfortable in hospital than at the practice. It's such a huge organization . . . You don't see the same person twice. They are a team, so just have to trust that the senior consultant reads the notes and that he would pick up on any problems.

THE NATURE OF TRUST RELATIONS BETWEEN HIP REPLACEMENT PATIENTS AND CLINICIANS IN SECONDARY CARE

The context of acute surgery in secondary care for our second case study offers a very different setting in which to explore patients' trust relationships with clinicians. In selecting this context, we proposed that patients undergoing elective hip surgery would have potentially very different relationships as they would not be familiar with the clinicians providing their care, unlike diabetes patients and their

GPs. In addition, the complexity of surgery reduces the ability of patients to act as expert patients, although as these were elective operations patients had the opportunity to become informed about the operation they were facing if they so wished. Similarly, patient choice meant that patients could express a preference regarding where to have the operation if they wanted. Although patients might have less scope to act as expert patients compared with those with long-term conditions, informed trust might still be relevant as the extent and nature of information clinicians provide may affect how much they trust the surgical team and the therapist and nursing care provided.

Figure 3.2 illustrates the trust relationships that hip surgery patients described as being important to them. The key relationship for patients was with the nurses on the wards and this was evidently much more important than their relationships with the medical team, physiotherapists and occupational therapists. Patients described how following surgery doctors and therapists would dip in and out of the ward to conduct a particular procedure or to check on progress, whereas the ward was run by the nurses and the bulk of care was provided by them and healthcare assistants.

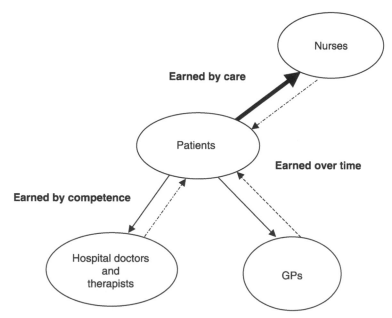

Figure 3.2   Trust relations between hip patients and clinicians

Hip patient 5: Hmm I don't think we have time for relationship with the doctors in there, in the hospital.
What do you mean by that?
Because um if they come round in the morning and um seeing to all the patients, they come and they ask you, 'How are you this morning?' 'I'm OK.' 'You feeling any pain?' 'Yes.' 'What kind of pain? Pain in your hip?' You know, and OK they will say, 'The nurses will see about you, will see to you, or anything for that.'
And that's it, the doctor is gone.

Patients' trust in clinicians was conditional in that it had to be earned and like the diabetes patients they distinguished between what they trusted different professionals to do. Patients' trust in nurses was earned by the quality of care they experienced, not just nurses' competence but their attitude and whether they were empathetic and caring in their approach, whereas it was the competence of the doctors and therapists which earned patients' trust. Although patients were grateful for the information provided to them about their operation and it helped reassure them, only one patient, a science lecturer, expressed informed trust, using information to calculate whether trust was warranted. She acted as an expert patient obtaining information from multiple sources and requiring information from the consultant before she would trust the team to proceed with surgery.

As with the diabetes case study, the need for mutual trust was expressed by hip surgery patients and hospital-based clinicians, with both identifying the need for clinicians to trust patients to follow clinical advice after discharge in terms of what activity should be undertaken to allow the new hip to bed in and avoid dislocation. However, in contrast to diabetes patients, the interdependence between patient and clinician was described less as a partnership and more in terms of a forced reliance which was not necessarily justified in the long term. Hospital clinicians expressed scepticism as to whether they could trust patients, due to experience of seeing patients not following medical advice or because they did not feel they knew them enough to be able to trust them:

Do you think doctors should trust patients, is that important?
Registrar: Yeah it's difficult that . . . I mean it would be nice to trust patients, but at the end of the day they're just somebody you've met for a couple of hours. You know, I know we expect it the other way but, you know. We expect to trust patients that they'll do what we say, that they won't put their legs in funny

positions so they dislocate things but, you know, there are a lot of um – you know, at the end of the day it is really hard to trust someone that you don't really know. I mean it is, isn't it?
Yeah, so really it doesn't matter, or you don't trust them as such?
I think the reality is I don't trust them, no.

Although questioned about their experience of secondary care, many patients raised the nature of their relationship with their GP, generally in favourable terms contrasting the trust that their GP had earned over time with the trust earned by the competence of hospital doctors. The limited relationship that patients had with the doctors on the wards created less opportunity for trust. In contrast, both senior and junior doctors considered it very important that patients trusted them, with the consultants suggesting that the detailed pre-operation assessment at which they agreed with the patient whether to undertake surgery was sufficiently lengthy to create trust between them.

Consultant 1: That is what I was saying about a doctor–patient relationship, I think you have got to sit down and spend time with the patient the first time you see them, so that you can generate a trusting relationship so that a patient will share their real problems with you and you and the patient then become the management team. The patient is never across the table from you, the patient has got problems and we are going to solve it together, the patient and I are going to solve it together. And you are going to do your best for them. I think that is really important.

Our two contrasting case studies show how trust relationships vary depending on the clinical condition and organizational setting. Opportunities for mutual trust between informed patients in partnership with clinicians are greater in primary care although not all patients want to take such an active role, preferring to have blind trust in their doctor. In both settings patient trust was usually conditional and had to be earned but it was not based upon information but experience in terms of the competence of the health professional and quality of care provided. Having examined the differences between trust relationships in two very diverse contexts, we now turn to consider common themes found in both case studies.

TYPES OF TRUST BETWEEN PATIENTS AND CLINICIANS

In both case studies the types of trust expressed by patients can be broadly categorized as either conditional or unconditional. In our theoretical framework we suggested that there might be a move away from the blind, unconditional trust associated with the traditionally paternalistic and deferent doctor–patient relationship towards a more questioning conditional trust. Our research suggests that there are still patients who simply assume they can trust healthcare professionals because of their professional status; such blind trust was expressed by a third of the diabetes and hip patients.

Unconditional 'blind' trust

One patient ascribed his unquestioning trust in doctors to his naturally trusting disposition while others proposed that it was a generational thing to hold their doctor in awe and recognized that it might now be considered old-fashioned.

When a patient says, 'Oh yes I trust my doctor,' what do you think, what do you understand by that?
Diabetes patient 9: Um well I – I just trust that they know what they're talking about . . . Um I mean if the doctor asks me to do something, then I usually try and do it, because I think well they're only doing it for my good. Um so I'm one of the old school, I'm afraid, I – I trust them implicitly.

The continuing unconditional trust in clinicians by some patients was confirmed by one of the GPs in the practice who said that reflected the kind of community the practice served. She did go on to recognize that people had changed and were more questioning and this was confirmed by the practice's receptionist who had worked at the practice for 27 years:

Do you think patients are less trusting of doctors now?
Receptionist: I think their expectations are different maybe. I think the media doesn't help obviously, and they read these horror stories and maybe the trust for GPs has gone, to what it was. I mean back when my Mum and Dad was younger obviously a doctor was God to them, you know, and I think that's gone, definitely. Yeah they don't put them on a pedestal like they used to.

Similarly, several of the nurses on the hospital wards thought patients were more questioning, to the extent of asking why they were having one type of prosthesis rather than another. One of the ward leaders recognized that blind trust was also a generational thing and was less common among younger patients:

> Ward leader 1: Occasionally you'll get somebody, you know, maybe some of the elderly still will say, 'Oh well, you know, I trust you doctor, I've got my life in your hands,' sort of thing. But um the younger people, you know, and the people up to or in their fifties are very much more challenging and questioning.

Our proposition that societal changes have created a more knowledgeable, less deferential patient population and in the process have changed the type of trust in healthcare professionals does appear to have been confirmed, at least among younger patients, and was echoed by one of the hip patients:

> Hip patient 6: When I was a kid in the sixties, there was pure blind trust. Now you must ask the question, 'Yeah but what happens?' or, 'Why?' or – and they can ask the same about you, you know what I mean. It should go both ways, you know what I mean. You shouldn't be arrogant or anything like that. . . . Because it was never open before, it was always a closed shop. Um – um now things are more open because everybody has to be more open, because that's the way society is like, you know.

One of the patients who expressed blind trust in his GP, as well as the nurses and doctors who had performed his hip operation, differentiated between GPs and hospital doctors, suggesting that while he trusted both of them, he had greater confidence in specialists because of their expert knowledge. For him confidence was linked to extent of knowledge whereas trust was associated with whether clinicians were doing their best for you.

Conditional trust

For the other patients interviewed, trust was more conditional; it either had to be earned or it was forced. Trust could be earned by clinicians providing reasonable information and explanations about their condition or a proposed treatment or through experience of their clinician's care. When diabetes patients were asked whether they would be willing to take a drug still under research, those that trusted their doctor implicitly were happy to take whatever was recommended whereas those who had more conditional trust would require much more information before doing so:

If your doctor wanted to treat you with a new drug being researched for diabetes, would you be willing to accept?
Diabetes patient 6: Not without a lot of questions. I wouldn't accept straight off, no, I'd ask a few questions.
What sort of questions?
Well, you know, how far has it been tested? Is it safe to be – to be taken? And what's been proved so far with it? You know, I would like to know.
Yeah, and if they didn't provide that, would you?
I think I'd decline. I don't think I would.

The competence of doctors and the quality of care provided by nurses were the main ways that hospital-based clinicians earned patients' trust. For some of the hip patients the reputation of a surgeon was enough to enable them to trust them and trust in the surgeon was then transferred to the surgical team. In contrast, the nurses tended to earn patients' trust by demonstrating their competence and quality of care:

Hip patient 6: The nurses are more hands on, so you tend to – you see how they react to certain things, and then you can see their professionalism . . . If – if there's – if there's a problem say with somebody else, you're watching and you see how they cope with that problem, and you think, 'Yeah, you know, there's not a problem there at all, yeah they know how to handle the situation, they know how to get over a problem like that.

This was confirmed by one of the ward leaders who said that nurses had to work harder to gain patients' trust. For most of the patients for whom trust was conditional, it was earned by their experience of care; only one hip patient expressed the 'informed trust' proposed in our theoretical model, whereby trust is warranted based on the information supplied by the clinician. Patient 12 was a science lecturer and she described how her trust in the surgeon was earned by him calling her at home and answering questions about the operation once she was informed she could trust him:

I wanted to talk to somebody. I rang his (the consultant's) um PA who said, 'Oh he's very, very busy now, I don't think you'll get to see him.' I was volunteering to come in and just have ten minutes or five minutes on the day when he was in surgery . . . And to my surprise and pleasure he phoned me at home that evening after 6.00, and I was able to have a reasonably long conversation, quarter of an hour, ten minutes or something.

Able to ask him questions about it, how many he'd done, what success rate, were there really any drawbacks? Final question: if you were in my position, would you have it done? And to which the answer was yes. I was completely happy with that. And I think, for me, that made a big difference.

While earned trust was similar for both diabetes and hip patients in that it was usually won through their experience of care, hip patients also talked about forced trust, where they felt they had to trust the doctor because they were ill.

Hip patient 6: I mean it's – actually I'm in their hands, I mean you've just got to trust them, haven't you? . . . But I mean when you're ill there's nothing else, there's nothing you can do really, I mean you have to trust your doctor.'

They reported they had to trust them to make the right decisions for their clinical care, even though they did not know them, because their life was in their hands. Such forced trust might be very typical in patients undergoing emergency treatment where they are not familiar with the clinicians and have no opportunity to assess whether trust is justified. Patients were less likely to express forced trust in nurses; trust in them was earned through experience, the competence they showed, the care they gave and their interest in the patient getting better. Forced trust was not expressed by diabetes patients and one of the GPs suggested that this was because in primary care patients ultimately have a choice in whether to accept their advice. One diabetes patient who had been a construction manager and was now actively retired did however question the relevance of trust at all. For him blind trust was inappropriate because doctors had let patients down by making errors; patients knew their bodies best and could access the information they needed on the Internet.

Diabetes patient 8: Um I don't really like this term 'trust'. I think – I think you want to feel they're doing their best, but the word trust is to implicitly think that they're right, and they're not always right.

DIMENSIONS OF TRUST

The literature suggests that trust is a multifaceted concept with a variety of dimensions including competence, confidentiality, acting in the other's interests and personal manner. In this research study, when patients were asked what trust meant to them the dominant dimension for them was the competence of clinicians and their ability to provide good care. All except 2 of the 20 patients interviewed talked about competence and for some patients it outweighed all other dimensions of trust, while others talked about competence in conjunction with other aspects such as confidentiality.

> *Right, so would you say that for you an important element of whether you trust a medical professional is how competent they are?*
> Diabetes patient 8: I think that's it entirely. I don't think it's um whether I like them or dislike them, or whether they've got a good bedside manner, sort of thing. I think it's whether or not you feel that they – they are um really competent in that particular thing.

Patients trusted doctors to have the skills and knowledge to know their job and make the right decisions. Competence encompassed communication skills as well as technical ability. Only one patient did not consider competence as being relevant to trust but at the same time he considered getting a good outcome as being important and this ultimately depends on clinical competence. For one patient the trust they had in a consultant was to do a specific job whereas their trust in their GP seemed more general and was based on familiarity as well as competence. Another patient talked about the lower trust they had for their GP compared with the specialist expertise of hospital doctors:

> Hip patient 17: Um sometimes with GPs I feel that they've got an awful lot to sort of take on board, therefore you need to be a little bit guarded, or wary of what they tell you sometimes. Whereas with a – once you get into hospital and you go to the people that know their subject, they've got full confidence like I did.

In contrast, only two patients, one from each case study, reported that confidentiality was important to trust, in particular being able to trust that information they gave would be kept confidential:

> Diabetes patient 3: It means to me that I can be very confidential with them and it won't go further than the four walls.

This dimension of trust either was taken for granted or just was not as significant as competence. Similarly, only five patients talked about altruism and the knowledge that clinicians act in the interests of their patients as being important to trust.

Hip patient 3: You trust them to do the very best for you to put your problem right, whatever it is.

On questioning patients, it appears that healthcare professionals' altruism is assumed; no patients thought that their doctors' or nurses' decisions were influenced by other than purely clinical considerations. It seemed to be taken for granted that their advice was based on what was best for the patient rather than being motivated by other factors such as financial considerations. In fact, one patient compared doctors favourably with bank managers whose motives could no longer be trusted.

Several patients talked about personal manner and honesty as being an important aspect of trust. The extent to which they liked their GP affected whether they trusted them.

Diabetes patient 8: Um I think it's a bit of a personal thing, that some people are trusting, you know. Some people say, 'Oh I trust in this um medicine I buy at the health shop,' or something like that. You know, I think that's a personal thing, somebody gets that feeling that they like their doctor, you know, they think they're a nice person.

Several of the hip patients talked about the personal manner of nurses and the extent to which they showed a caring attitude as being important as to whether they trusted them. Honesty was also raised by one of the hip patients:

Hip patient 4: You knew what was going on all the time, there was nothing done behind your back – well it might have been, but not to my knowledge. But they kept me in the picture about everything like, so I couldn't wish for anything else, not really.

HOW TRUST IS BUILT AND LOST

How trust can be built or lost depends on a patient's understanding of trust, so that if a patient needs trust to be earned through competence, then effective technical and communication skills will earn their trust and incompetence will lose it. For most patients trust was created by their experience of care and the clinician's personal manner, technical competence and communication skills. Communication is a key mechanism for trust building, being open with patients and honest with the information provided helps to generate trust.

What encourages you to trust your doctor or nurse?
Diabetes patient: Just the things that they impart to you, you know, they sit you down and tell you. You tell them and then they diagnose and they sit you down and tell you. So I mean that gives me trust, that they're taking the trouble to explain what is wrong.

Similarly, in the hip case study communication was valued partly because it displays a clinician's competence, and partly because it offers reassurance. The specialist technical knowledge of hospital doctors increased one patient's trust in them compared with his GP.

Clinicians in both clinical settings echoed patients' views in suggesting that personal manner, honesty and the respect they showed patients would build trust in them.

Lead diabetes nurse: I think it's because we're honest with them whether it's good or bad. I think we're honest and don't try to fob them off with some, you know 'Oh there, there' or paint a rosy picture – and I think they respect that and they trust us because they know we're telling the truth.

Personal manner involved not just being friendly but finding out about each patient's background in order to try to tailor advice to meet their preferences and needs:

Occupational therapist: Um simple things like body language and, you know, um having a chat with them, getting a bit of background, and trying to gain their patient – their sort of individual perspective on issues, and just trying to kind of work with them to um sort of er set up, devise recommendations that work for them. And um sort of reasoning as well, clinical reasoning, explaining the basis of the recommendation, and giving them information.

In the hospital setting nurses also identified the importance of cleanliness as being important in building patients' trust in the hospital and nursing staff. They observed that patients judge the quality of care and the overall experience of their hospital stay by the standards of hygiene and cleanliness of the ward.

Ward leader 2: From the time that the patients come in you start building that trust, just by the way you welcome them, um the efficiency, the organization, you know, just having a clean and tidy ward just shows, you know, how much. People will – you know, I sit there myself and I think, 'Oh God, look at that, look at this.' And, you know, having toilets clean, you know, it's all in the media. And patients are so observant.

Interestingly, patients did not report familiarity or the length of time that they had known a clinician as being important in building trust, although a number of the hospital doctors considered that GPs had an advantage because they may have had many years to get to know a patient. It seems that how patients are treated and whether their experience of a consultation in a practice or on the ward is positive is much more important than familiarity in creating trust between a patient and a clinician. This is important given the increasingly team-based approach to patient care, both within secondary and primary care. Some of the diabetes patients preferred to wait for an appointment with their personal GP rather than see another GP in the practice but this seemed to be because they were familiar with their history rather than because they did not trust the other doctors.

The role of information in creating trust was also subtle. Information per se did not build trust, except in the case of one of the hip patients who wanted performance data on the number of successful operations the consultant had completed. Instead, information was valued because it suggested that clinicians were being honest and open with patients and it also showed them some respect. Performance data such as a hospital's star rating did not appear to influence a patient's trust in a hospital. None of the patients mentioned it spontaneously and when asked by the interviewer whether this contributed to their trust in a hospital all but one patient responded in the negative, with many dismissing such information as lacking credibility because figures have been manipulated to meet political targets.

Although most patients considered it important that clinicians trusted them as well as vice versa, very few had considered what might build trust in them as patients. Some suggested that trust in them is engendered by them being honest with their clinician, particularly if they have not followed their advice. For primary care clinicians whether they could trust patients' ability to self-manage depended on a patient's competence in terms of their understanding of their condition.

What would patients have to do to make you trust their ability to self-manage their condition?
Salaried GP: I'd want them to understand what their condition was and understand its implications for their health. And understand what the medication was trying to do and ideally to

remember what is the name for it. And obviously to be fairly sharp. I mean I think there are some people where they just don't have the intellect to cope with that.

While patients were quite ready to talk about how trust is built and were clear that it did need to be constructed, they generally found it harder to talk about how trust is lost. Complaints, the NHS's financial problems and negative media coverage were not mentioned by patients. Instead, loss of trust revolved around the patient experience and related to specific bad experiences of care such as an unsuccessful operation, or where medication was changed without any beneficial outcome, or where a clinician had been rude or disrespectful.

> Diabetes patient: Well if I went there sort of now, and he started mucking about with my tablets, or changing this, that or the other, and it didn't have any difference or any benefit, any difference, you know, it wasn't – it made things worse instead of better or something like that, I mean that is what would er make me lose trust.

> Hip patient 4: But through him just walking out in the middle of trying to tell us, and no follow up, no letter or nothing, then I – I – you know, I might be wrong, but if he'd have built up a trust then I'd have turned round and said, 'Well yeah, that's fair enough, he knows what he's on about, you know, he's doing what he can.' But he didn't, he just got very abrupt and that was it. So straight away I had no trust in him, and if I'd had to see him again I'd have probably turned round and said, 'No I'm not going to bother.'

Such negative experiences of care, either suffered directly or indirectly by friends or family, could lead to a complete loss of trust. One hip patient talked about how they had lost trust in a GP because they had not been confidential about the patient's illness. Having lost that patient's trust they would never see that doctor again:

> Hip patient 5: But um I wouldn't trust him than I can throw him.
> *Hmm, hmm.*
> And even if I'm dying I wouldn't go to him.
> *Why?*
> Because um he was – you couldn't trust him, because you would tell – he would tell somebody else your problem. You get me?

Patients were sceptical about the influence of the media on their trust in clinicians and healthcare institutions. While they recognized that it might make them slightly wary before coming into hospital, they also recognized that their own experience of care had left them no cause for complaint and that the media tended only to report negative experiences. Similarly, instances of foul play such as Howard Shipman were dismissed by most patients as a one-off or highly unusual, and had not affected patient trust in doctors.

> Hip patient 17: Well I suppose there's um – there's all sorts of people like Shipman in all walks of life, and it's just extremely unlucky those poor ladies um, or there might have been one or two men wouldn't it, but mostly elderly ladies had to encounter a man like that. And it's got to be a very rare thing surely, yeah.

HIGH TRUST AND LOW TRUST BEHAVIOUR

Prior to our empirical investigation we suggested a number of behaviours that might be indicative of high and low trust (see Chapter 2, Table 2.5 on p. 53). Following our interviews with patients we have refined this list to include patient-identified behaviours, as shown in Table 3.1. A number of patients suggested that their willingness to follow the doctor's advice was a sign of their trust in them and they did not check their recommendations with other sources.

> *Do you ever check the advice that you get at all? You know, when they give you advice, do you ever check it?*
> Diabetes patient 10: No. With who – with whom?
> *Well sometimes people will look in a book, or younger ones nowadays have the Internet, you know.*
> No, no I don't never um.
> *You never check?*
> I don't never um doubt their word.

The hip patients also exhibited high trust behaviour; none asked for a second opinion prior to surgery and only one patient checked the advice received on the Internet prior to surgery. In fact, one patient made it clear that he considered it the surgeon's job to decide on the type of operation required, he was the expert and ultimately as a taxpayer the patient was paying for him to make those decisions. Patients' reluctance to participate in decision-making and

Table 3.1 High and low trust behaviour as identified by patients

High trust behaviour	Described by patients	Low trust behaviour
Willingness to divulge information	X	Information is withheld
Passive, deferential role	X	Questioning, possibly sceptical role
Forgive errors and mistakes		Errors result in blame, possibly complaints and choice of alternative provider
Low anxiety	X	High anxiety
Hygiene left to hospital staff	X	Patients bring personal disinfectant into hospital
Waiting to see a specific clinician	X	Avoidance of a particular clinician following errors
Advice is accepted willingly	X	Request for a second opinion or alternative source of treatment sought

willingness to accept clinical advice without questioning was confirmed by one of the research fellows in the hospital:

> Research fellow 1: So in the UK they don't, so you still will, in a clinic where you're consenting people for surgery let's say, you will still have a good 40 per cent of them saying, 'Oh don't tell me about the complications doctor, I don't want to know, just get on with it.' You know, and you say, 'Well no, you have to know, because of this.' And they say, 'Well no, I don't want to know.' And then you just have to document that, that the patient was offered the information.

This high trust behaviour extended to patients indicating that they would be willing to participate in a research study, testing a new medication for diabetes or a new surgical prosthesis, although patients made the proviso that their doctor needed to believe it would be of benefit to them and that it needed to be safe. One patient suggested that his lack of anxiety prior to the operation was an indicator of his trust in the surgical team.

> Patient 17: When you went to the theatre you were ready for the

operation and um, you know, I didn't feel overly nervous or anything like that, I just felt, 'OK I'm going to have my operation now,' slightly sort of excited about it.

Given the high trust in clinicians that patients reported, they found it difficult to describe occasions when they had acted out of low trust. However, when talking critically about locum GPs or other hospital specialists, it was evident that patients had behaved in ways that we had proposed. Questioning of clinical advice was reported by one patient who was getting side-effects from a medication for her diabetes. She refused to accept the advice of a locum doctor that she had to put up with the side-effects. Not trusting the locum's advice, she saw her own doctor a little later and was able to resolve the problem, confirming in her view that she was correct not to have trusted the other doctor. However, questioning per se is not necessarily indicative of low trust. The salaried GP thought that patients were generally more questioning not because they distrusted their doctor, but simply because they wanted more information. In fact, in both case studies only about a third of patients could be classified as wishing to be actively involved in the management of their condition. None of the diabetes patients checked the advice they had been given by their clinician on the Internet.

Similarly, the majority of the hip patients did not question the advice from the hospital doctors, nurses or therapists. In fact, one patient suggested that doctors might lose trust in patients if it was found they were checking their advice with another doctor. This lack of questioning may be age-related as all the patients were over 50 or might be due to relief that their condition was being dealt with. Patients were aware of the Internet as a useful source of information but they did not use it to check their doctor's advice. One patient explained that their daughter had used an Internet chat room to find out about the surgery to explain to her children what was happening to their grandparent but the patient herself had not found the information useful. The hospital was the key source of information and provided sufficient advice for patients:

> Patient 17: Oh I think she (my daughter) probably looked up one or two of the things. But no, I didn't rely on the computer or anything, I got all the information I wanted from the hospital anyway, so it was fine.

Limited questioning may also be indicative of the complex nature of hip surgery; at least one of the patients had taken a more active role over a less serious health problem. He had questioned his GP's recommendation to start anti-hypertension drugs, insisting that he had a monitor to check that his blood pressure was abnormal away from the surgery before being willing to start medication. The response of the patients interviewed may also not be typical of hip patients. One of the ward leaders reported that patients were becoming more questioning and were increasingly using the Internet to check information:

> Ward leader 1: Because they've got all this information off the Internet. And they also can get information about their consultant, in many instances, over the Internet, because some of them have got websites.
> *Do they use them?*
> Oh yeah they do. And one, when I was doing a clinic, you know, an extra clinic outside my work, um with a shoulder consultant, and he was actually seeing somebody about total knee replacement, because he actually did do knees as well, and this man said, 'Oh well it says on the web that you only do shoulders, so what are you looking at my knee for?' You know, and that did not go down well. Um so, yeah, they're much – they're, in a way, much more informed, but they're not.

Low trust is much more likely to result in avoidance of a clinician than active complaining. When the practice, a GP, or the local hospital may have made an error or provided inadequate care, the patient's response was to avoid that particular person or practice because their trust in their competence had been eroded, rather than complaining.

> *I mean just finishing on that question about the surgery, did you feel like complaining at all about the practice?*
> Diabetes patient 8: Um well I did, but at the time I didn't really feel like doing it. I felt like dying at the time, I felt really bad. You know, um it wasn't something that er I wanted anything to do with at the time. And I was so pleased with the advice I was getting at the acute hospital that I wrote the surgery off.

The senior receptionist confirmed that this was a pattern of behaviour displayed regularly by patients:

> Um it's when you get someone who says, 'Oh I don't want to see that doctor again,' and you think, 'What's going on here?'

And does that happen?
It does, yes it does, more so today than when I first started.
And what do you think that's about?
I think again it's the rush, it's, you know, the time limit they've
got, the 10 minutes each appointment, they're afraid to run too
much over, which is understandable.

Similarly, lack of complaints by hospital patients does not necessarily mean that they trust clinicians or a particular hospital. One
patient who had had a bad experience at another hospital and did
not trust the doctors there still had not complained.

Whether patients would be willing to find an alternative provider
if they lost trust depended on how active they were in managing their
condition. Patients who were passive in managing their diabetes said
they would be reluctant to move practice if they lost trust in a particular doctor because of the convenience of the local practice and
their ability to see another GP at the same practice if necessary. Even
when a patient had had a bad experience at the practice, with a
serious condition going undiagnosed for several months, he was still
unwilling to move due to the effort involved and a concern that his
notes might get lost in the process. In contrast, two patients who
were very active in managing their condition were more ready to
criticize and potentially move practice or use private healthcare if
they were not satisfied with the NHS.

Patient 5: If I don't feel that I'm getting what I want then I will
go private. But not for diabetes.
What would cause you to lose your trust in them? Well, if they
didn't respond in a reasonable way in a reasonable time. If I felt
that I wasn't going to get that service then I would go private.
And yes I would change my GP if I lost trust in them.

These more active diabetes patients were more likely to seek a second
opinion if they were not satisfied with a hospital consultant.

A lot of the strategies open to patients who did not trust a GP
were not available to those undergoing hip surgery. In general, they
were not in a position to avoid clinicians or to be able to question
them in detail about their operation due to its complexity. Alternative behaviour indicative of low trust included patients expressing
fear and anxiety prior to going into hospital for an operation. This
anxiety tended to be linked less to concerns about the surgical or
technical competence of staff and more to fears about acquiring an
infection during their stay. Lack of trust in a hospital's standards

of hygiene caused some patients to bring their own bottles of disinfectant with them.

> Ward leader 2: Yeah I mean many of them come in with their little bottles of er – of disinfectant and stuff, um and they're quite hot on it, they're hot on watching nurses wash their hands. You know, we have audits where infection control come around, and they'll discuss it with the patients, and one of the first things they'll say is, 'Well that nurse never washed her hands.' The thing is, a lot of them don't see past that room, they don't see that the nurse might come into the clinical room and wash her hands there, um so a lot of it can be misleading. But they sit there, they watch, they have high expectations, they've heard of MRSA, half of them don't know what it is, and they've heard of clostridium, they've heard of Norwalk, and a lot of it is all just words to them, but they've heard them, and it's all going on in their mind, I should think. So by seeing the nurse wash their hands every time, the trust builds up.

Even though patients voiced concern over the cleanliness of NHS hospitals, they would not necessarily seek private treatment if they did not trust the NHS. They had heard stories of people experiencing problems with their care in private facilities and did not equate 'going private' as being a better or more trustworthy option.

BENEFITS AND DISADVANTAGES OF TRUST

As reported in other research studies into the effects of trust, patients identified better health outcomes as being the key benefit of trust. Trust encouraged full disclosure of health problems, enabling symptom control and more effective management of their diabetes:

> *I mean is it important that they trust you?*
> Diabetes patient 6: Yeah I think so. I mean if I'm not giving them the right information then they can't give me the right cure so.

It also encouraged patients to access health services. Several hip patients suggested that trust indirectly promoted better patient outcomes because it encouraged good teamworking among clinicians:

> Hip patient 4: I think it's just an overall package really, that um if they all trust each other they're going to make each other's

job a lot easier, and hopefully the condition will heal a lot sooner and more efficiently.

One of the nurses thought trust promoted better outcomes because patients were more confident in their ability to cope and continue with their rehabilitation at home. As in Dibben and Lena's (2003) research trust appears to be fostered when clinicians build up a patient's sense of self-competence.

Several patients talked about the benefits of mutual trust where they trust their clinician and their clinician trusts them. For one patient this meant that he only sought an appointment when there was a real problem, ensuring more efficient use of clinical time. Other patients said that there was better concordance with treatment when there was mutual trust:

> *Is it important that you trust your doctor or your nurse?*
> Diabetes patient 9: Um yes, to me it is, yes I think it is important that you do trust them, yeah.
> *But I'm going to ask you why?*
> Well it's er, I don't know, if I didn't trust them, I mean you're not likely to do what they're getting you to do, or asking you to do. So um I mean I trust what they're saying is the correct thing, and I – I try to go along with what they ask me to do, or tell me to do, or whatever.

One of the patients in the hip study also recognized the mutual benefits of trust:

> Hip patient 3: Because I think if you haven't got trust then um neither of you are really going to benefit. You're not going to benefit from their experience and expertise, and they're not going to benefit from you trying to help them by giving them as much information, and doing as much as possible what they advise you to do.

Patients in both case studies found it difficult to identify disadvantages to trust. Only one diabetes patient saw any potential drawback to trusting their clinician in that they might not question their advice or the information given and that might lead to poorer outcomes.

> Diabetes patient: I don't know that absolute sort of um faith in the doctor is always a good thing. I think you've also got to er use your – you know, only you know about yourself. And also, over time, you learn about what's wrong with you, what's wrong

with yourself, and what sort of treatment, you know. To the doctor you're a stranger.
Could it (too much trust) be harmful, do you think?
I think it could be, because you could sort of sus that the doctor had given the wrong – given you the wrong information, whereas perhaps if you er had reason not to think er that the doctor was right, and you asked for a second opinion, the second opinion may be the one that er could save your life for you then. (laughs)

Only one patient discounted any clinical benefit of trust, except for people with mental health problems:

Do you see potentially some disadvantages if people trust too much?
Hip patient 8: Yes I think there is, you know, I think there is some disadvantages in – er in complete – in complete trust. I think it said in that um paper 'would you feel – would it make you feel better, or would it make you feel – would you get better quicker?' or something like that, if you had trust . . . Um only, I think, if you've got some mental problem, you know. If it's a purely medical problem, I don't think it makes any difference whatsoever.

Not surprisingly, clinicians did not identify any disadvantages in patients trusting them. Instead, one of the GPs raised the problem of how patients could recognize trustworthy sources of information. She considered that some of the information provided by the Internet might reduce patients' trust in their GPs if it offered conflicting advice.

CONCLUSIONS

The findings of our research suggest that trust relations between patients and clinicians are influenced by organizational and clinical context but that there are as many similarities as there are differences between clinical settings. Social changes may have encouraged patients to be more questioning and less deferential but there are still patients, both in primary and secondary care, who prefer to trust unconditionally in their doctor or nurse. Increasingly, patients' trust in clinicians is conditional and is earned by their experience of care and the nature of their relationship with their clinician. There does appear to be greater interdependence between patients and clinicians requiring increased mutual trust but there are differences between the clinical contexts. In primary care the clinician–patient relationship can be characterized as more of a partnership, whereby patients may be willing to wait to see the GP or nurse who has earned their trust and is familiar with their history. In the secondary care setting, mutual trust can be earned but it is also forced; due to the acute nature of their condition patients have to trust the surgical team to a certain extent as their life is literally in their hands. Similarly, with shorter lengths of stay clinicians have to trust that patients will continue with their rehabilitation at home as advised.

Patients, irrespective of whether they have a long-term condition or are having elective surgery, prioritize competence as the key dimension of trust and appear to assume that clinicians will act in patients' best interests and will keep their clinical information confidential. Trust is built through competence and communication; every interaction between clinician and patient appears to provide an opportunity for clinicians to display openness, honesty and an empathetic personal manner as well as technical competence. We identified only a small number of instances when patients appeared to act on informed trust, whereby they decided whether trust was warranted based on the information provided; instead information was valued because of the openness and respect it indicated for patients. Performance data and media reports did not influence patients' trust in a particular clinician or institution; rather their views were shaped by personal experience either directly by themselves or indirectly by friends or family. Just as trust is built based on personal experiences it can be lost in a similar way after a poor experience of care. When trust has been lost patients in primary care were more likely to take steps to avoid the clinician in question rather than complain or change practice altogether. Such strategies were not open to patients in secondary care; for hip surgery patients their level of anxiety prior to their operation and whether they brought in bottles of disinfectant were indicators of their trust in the competence of the surgical team and the ward staff.

For the majority of patients interviewed trust was still very relevant to their relationship with clinicians. All patients, except one diabetes patient who had had a bad experience of care at the practice, talked at length of the importance of trust. Trust was needed if they were to provide personal information about their health and if they were then to heed the advice given by their doctor, nurse or therapist. This suggests that trust between patients and clinicians is not only important for patient outcomes and the doctor–patient relationship but is important for the NHS more broadly if patients are to access and use health services appropriately and effectively. In the next chapter we turn to examine how trust between healthcare professionals affects the effectiveness of health service provision.

4

TRUST BETWEEN CLINICIANS

In contrast to the substantial literature on patient trust in doctors and nurses, studies that have investigated the nature of trust between clinicians and its impact on the effectiveness of healthcare provision are relatively sparse. In this first investigation of inter-clinician trust in the UK NHS we report on the nature of trust relations that exist between a range of health professionals working in the two case study settings of a general practice and an acute hospital. We examine whether and how trust relations are changing as a result of new ways in which health services are being provided and we consider the effects of such changes on patient trust in clinicians and in healthcare institutions.

THE NATURE OF TRUST RELATIONS BETWEEN CLINICIANS IN PRIMARY CARE

In the last decade UK general practice has undergone considerable change in how services are delivered to patients. The days of sole practitioners providing continuous 24-hour care to their personal list of patients have been largely consigned to history. Today, most surgeries are multi-partner practices with much of chronic care management delegated to nurse practitioners, practice nurses and healthcare assistants. Practices have largely opted out of providing out-of-hours care and this is now the responsibility of local primary care trusts and out-of-hours cooperatives. In Chapter 2 we suggested that these changes in healthcare delivery may have created the need for new trust relations as GPs and nurses share the care of their patients. Instead of trust being dependent on an individual's position, such as a partner's general practitioner status, trust may increasingly have to be earned both between GPs and with other clinical members of the practice.

In our general practice case study there was a network of trust relations, as illustrated in Figure 4.1. GPs talked about their trust in hospital doctors and the practice nurses as well as their fellow GPs and the nurses referred to their trust in other nurses, the healthcare assistants and the GPs. In all such relationships, with the exception of those between GPs and hospital doctors, informants described how trust needed to be two-way; it was important that nurses felt they could trust the GPs as much as vice versa. The loss of personal lists meant that GPs could no longer operate as autonomous healthcare providers; patient care was shared between GPs and responsibility for much chronic disease management was delegated to the nurses within the practice, under the leadership of the diabetes lead nurse who had agreed a management protocol with the lead GP for diabetes. This meant that while GPs were still responsible for diagnosing diabetes and prescribing appropriate treatment, the

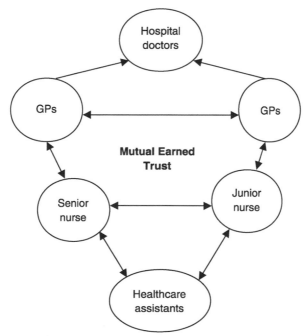

Figure 4.1   Trust relations between clinicians in the primary care setting

ongoing monitoring of a patient's condition was the remit of the practice nurses. In this particular practice relationships between clinicians could be characterized as being typically of mutual respect; clinicians had similar values and ideals and communication between them was reported to be good.

The shared care approach for diabetes patients created the need for greater trust between health professionals but it also provided the key mechanism by which trust could be earned. All clinicians reported that patient reports and their experience of care provided by another clinician within the practice were the main way in which they decided whether trust in a colleague was merited.

> Salaried GP: I can see when I see patients coming through that have been seen by other doctors, I don't question the judgements that they've made. I don't question their choice of treatment plan.

The practice nurses suggested that in their management of patients it was important for them to show awareness of their own competencies and to be cautious not to overstep their ability in order to earn the trust of the GPs in the practice.

> *Is it important that you trust the GPs and the GPs trust you?*
> Practice nurse: Oh yeah it's imperative really. And hopefully they do. I think you know, you have to be confident but also, um, you have to know your own abilities and be cautious. So confident with caution, I think that's really from the nursing point of view what the GPs are looking for.

While time is typically cited as a key factor in building trust, nurse trust in GPs depended on the competence of the practitioner as much as their personal knowledge of them over time.

> Diabetes nurse: I think it's because I've got to know them as a person, so I know them better, so I can see the way their mind works. And it's like the more you get to know somebody and if you get a rapport with them, then you do trust them. Then there are other doctors who I don't know so well but their clinical judgement is absolutely spot on, clinically they are absolutely fantastic . . . And then there are others, you know, where you think well if I send this patient there that might not be the best doctor for them to see with that condition, because their expertise is somewhere else.

Between nurses trust had again to be earned and was based on the clinical competence of their colleagues which was assessed over time. This was important for senior nurses' trust in junior nurses and for junior nurses and healthcare assistants' trust in the senior nurses; how senior nurses responded to a junior's queries about what to do about certain clinical problems helped foster trust between the nurses.

There were only two relationships where more traditional trust relations could be seen, between GPs and hospital doctors and between healthcare assistants and the practice nurses. The latter exhibited a more hierarchical relationship with healthcare assistants being delegated particular tasks which were closely supervised. Trust was dependent on how the healthcare assistants responded to direct questions about the treatment they had given patients. Trust relations between GPs and hospital doctors appear to be undergoing a process of change. Whereas previously GPs may have sought and sometimes still did seek to refer to a named consultant, with trust in them being based on their reputation and the seniority of their position, increasingly they were referring to a hospital team. In such circumstances trust was less individualized and related more to trust in a given secondary care team. Whether this was earned depended on their patients' experience of care and also the quality of communication between the hospital doctor and the GP.

What makes you trust a doctor in the acute hospital?
Executive partner: I think experience of them, which gets harder the older you are somehow, because it's a long time since I worked in a hospital so a lot of the names that I refer to now I don't know personally . . . so until I've seen what they do with a few of my patients, I may not know, unless I've heard of their reputation through somebody else.

Changes in healthcare delivery in terms of the loss of personal GP lists and the increasing nurse management of long-term conditions have resulted in the need for a more shared care approach to patient care in general practice. As a result trust between clinicians in the primary care team is more relevant than it has ever been. However, the shared care approach also provides the mechanism for building trust as GPs and nurses see how patients have been managed by their colleagues.

THE NATURE OF TRUST RELATIONS BETWEEN CLINICIANS IN SECONDARY CARE

The team of clinicians who provide care to patients undergoing elective hip surgery is significantly larger and more complex than clinical relationships found in primary care. The core surgical team comprises a medical team and a nursing team, and a physiotherapist if a named individual has been assigned to a given team, as illustrated in Figure 4.2.

Outside this core team clinicians may interact with a variety of health professionals based in other departments in order to provide care to a particular patient. This includes other doctors based in the medical as opposed to the surgical directorate as well as support services such as pathology and radiology and therapists in occupational therapy, physiotherapy and social work. When discussing trust between clinicians, informants referred to relationships within the core surgical team; these were the key relationships where trust or the lack of it was most important. Informants suggested that trust between the nurses and doctors in a surgical team needed to be mutual and that it was earned through experience over time by the honesty, reliability and competence of their colleagues. Trust between nurses and trust between doctors also appeared to be conditional and earned through experience but elements of status trust were evident whereby untrained nurses or junior doctors trusted their more senior colleagues due to their greater experience and seniority.

> Junior registrar: If it's someone senior to me, I tend to always mentally – I've got it, you know, maybe it's just the way I've been brought up and that, I've kind of got it in my head, the way I am, if it's someone senior they know more than me, they're right. . . . I think I, you know, if my boss said he trusted someone else's judgement, that's what I'd go along with.

Although the organizational setting of secondary care is more complex with a greater number of interactions between a greater variety of health professionals, our theoretical framework suggested that we might find a similar shift from peer-based trust, whereby a clinician trusts another clinician based on their position within the medical hierarchy, to earned trust where trust depends on the clinical competence of a colleague. We suggested that this may have been stimulated by changes in the nursing profession, whereby nurses are no longer willing to act as handmaidens to the medical profession,

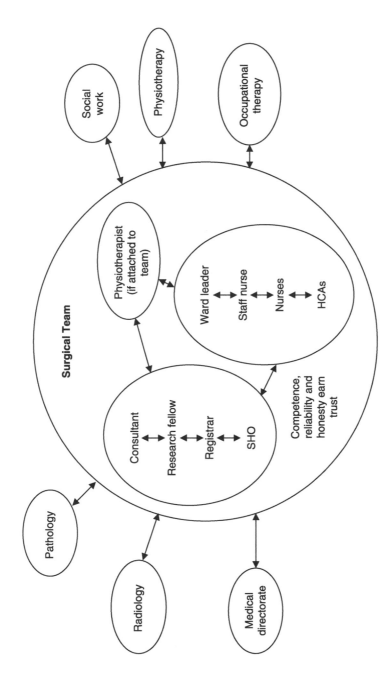

Figure 4.2 Trust relations between clinicians within a surgical team in an acute hospital

and by the multidisciplinary team-based approach to patient care whereby clinicians other than doctors such as occupational therapists and physiotherapists have input into determining whether a patient is fit for discharge. Such changes in healthcare delivery did indeed appear to have created new more mutual trust relations between clinicians in secondary care but another change in how healthcare is organized emerged as a key influence on trust relationships between clinicians. The European Working Time Directive has since 2004 required a significant reduction in doctors' working hours, and in order to be compliant hospitals in the UK have reformed their shift system for medical staff. For many of the doctors interviewed in our second case study, the introduction of the new shift system has made trust all the more important but it was not trust earned through experience or based on personal knowledge of another doctor but forced trust, as much in systems as in people.

> Senior house officer: Because as in shift system, like if I am not working on a week and somebody is looking after my patients, or I am away on leave and somebody is looking after my patients, I think trust is quite important.

> Fellow: You have to work in teams more now just because hours have changed. So in the past it was, you know, you're here all the time. Whereas you're not here all the time, so you have to have good hand-overs, and you have to have trusting that this system works.

Trust was described as fundamental to the effective working of the surgical team but the sense from informants was that this was created in spite of the system of healthcare delivery rather than thanks to how healthcare was organized. There was a sense among the doctors interviewed that the new shift system had forced them to trust more in their colleagues, including those not known to them, making trust less individual and personal. In subsequent sections we examine the types of trust shown in both case studies and identify how trust is built and lost, what constitutes high and low trust behaviour, and the impact of trust on the effectiveness of clinical care.

TYPES OF TRUST BETWEEN CLINICIANS

In the theoretical framework described in Chapter 2, we suggested that there may have been a shift in the type of trust shown between clinicians from one based on status, where junior nurses or doctors would automatically trust senior colleagues because of their seniority, greater experience and position within the medical or nursing hierarchy, to a more conditional type of trust which had to be earned by the competence of the clinician. In both case studies we found that conditional trust was prevalent between clinicians and that it had to be earned over time and was dependent on the honesty, reliability and competence of clinical colleagues.

Conditional trust earned over time

In primary care, trust is earned indirectly as it is largely dependent on their patients' experience of treatment by a colleague as reported by patients, or as indicated in their medical record or in correspondence with secondary care.

In terms of trusting that they're competent to do that, how do you judge that, if you like?
Practice nurse: Questioning and um, you know, you refer the patients and then they'll come back to, and you can see the kind of um treatment that they've been given by them. And also the patient will tell you. I mean there's no better person to tell you what they like than the patient. I know they tell the doctor if they're not happy as well with you. So I mean, you know, patients, they'll equally sing your praises, or will equally say when you're going wrong.

A clinician may initially assume that they may be able to trust a colleague but only experience will show whether trust is warranted. In the case of referral to secondary care, if GPs lose trust in a hospital doctor they will simply not refer patients to them.

Executive GP: I suppose there is an assumption that if someone's got to be a relatively senior doctor in a trust, in a secondary care, then they should have a level of competence. But there are some consultants that I would avoid referring to.

For hospital-based clinicians trust is equally conditional but is earned more directly through working with clinical colleagues, watching the way they go about certain clinical tasks, how they treat patients, and the type of questions they ask. This is particularly relevant for trust between doctors as medical rotation means that junior doctors change on a regular basis. Through such experience senior clinicians gauge whether a colleague is honest, competent and reliable and therefore trustworthy and junior doctors learn what is expected of them.

Some of the medical practitioners talked about initially assuming they could trust a fellow doctor, both in terms of junior doctors trusting other more senior colleagues due to their senior position, and senior doctors trusting junior staff on the basis that problems would have already been picked up.

> Registrar: A lot of people don't choose their junior staff, they're given to you, and you just hope that the problem may have been picked up earlier on if someone is not trustworthy. So you do kind of assume it.

But informants then went on to describe how medical colleagues earned their trust through experience in terms of how doctors went about things.

> Registrar: And just the way that they go about things, you can kind of gauge, you know, whether someone's done this before by the sort of routine they do for certain tasks.

Experience of another clinician's way of working will enable their colleagues to know how they might respond in a given situation and to be reassured (or not) that they will provide the same standard of care as you would. For all clinicians being aware of the limits of their clinical competence and recognizing what they don't know were very important in determining whether colleagues considered that you were a safe and reliable pair of hands who could be trusted.

> Junior registrar: Now um most people are alright to rely on, because most of us know our limitations, you know, and if any-thing we're a bit more keen to call [a senior doctor] than not call nowadays, so we know our limitations. And as long as you're a person who knows your limitations, I don't think you're dan-gerous as a doctor.

> Registrar: I mean you kind of gauge from the questions people ask and the – you know, I think that's the main thing, the ques-tions they ask, because that reflects where they're uncertain about things, so you kind of gauge from that.

Nurse trust in other nurses was also earned over time and depended on their nursing colleague's competence.

Staff nurse: Trust isn't an automatic thing, you can't just immediately go and trust somebody, you've got to build a relationship with them. You've got to be able to communicate with that person, you know, um and then out of that, you know, you find out, yes they are, you know, competent at doing this, this and this. You know, and then you know that you could go and ask them, and you know that you can trust them enough to go and do the job.

Competence was important in terms of earning trust for all levels of clinician; one healthcare assistant said that there were only certain people that she would trust to get a patient up with her after a difficult hip revision. Likewise, physiotherapy assistants earned the trust of the senior physiotherapist over time as they showed their competence. As a result she had lower trust in new staff and supervised them more closely.

Physiotherapist: So you build up your trust in somebody in the time and experience that you've had working with them. And in terms of new members of staff, I probably molly-coddle or just, you know, don't deliberately look over their shoulder but, you know, you keep an eye on how they're managing with their workload, are they managing to see all their patients, or do they have their personal time to do their CPD etc.?

Reliability was a key issue for trust to develop between doctors, nurses and therapists. Trust is earned by people doing things you ask them to and could build trust between professions as well as within professions.

Staff nurse: Because at the end of the day, they [doctors] come in and they say, 'We want this, this and this done,' well if you don't do it then they're not going to trust you to do it for them again.

Conditional trust which is forced

When discussing trust relations between clinicians, informants in both case studies were clear that trust was important and that it had to be earned over time. In contrast, when discussing clinicians' trust in patients there was a marked contrast between the two case studies. In the hip case studies the clinicians considered it very important that patients trusted them because surgery was such a major event. But they also recognized that they needed to trust that patients were being honest about their symptoms prior to surgery and their ability to cope at home after the operation and that they would do their rehabilitation exercises after being discharged.

> Occupational therapist: It's important that you're trusting the information that you're actually being given is correct. Because that obviously forms a big part of your assessment in terms of somebody's ability to cope.
> *Do some patients lie?*
> I wouldn't say lie, but I think sometimes it can be very difficult for patients if they're desperate to get back home, to actually say, 'Yeah – no I think everything's OK, I can cope.' Um I don't think it – I wouldn't describe it as lying, but I think it's very difficult for a patient who is so desperate to get home. And perhaps from all other professionals' points of view, from a medical point of view they could go, but from social problems it would be an unsafe discharge, I think that's very difficult for patients.

However, despite recognizing this need for mutual trust, many of the clinicians suggested that they were forced to trust their patients and their willingness to follow their rehabilitation advice following discharge. If a patient was keen to be discharged and clinicians agreed, given the constant pressure to ensure short lengths of stay, they were forced to trust that the patient would comply with clinical advice. However, some clinicians went on to voice a lack of trust in patients following their instructions once they were home.

The chronic nature of diabetes and the extent of influence that patients have in deciding how to manage the condition created a different type of relationship in primary care where clinicians did not feel they were forced to trust in patients. When discussing whether they could or needed to trust patients, several GPs suggested that this was not necessary given the nature of the doctor–patient relationship in primary care. Although GPs and nurses could advise and agree on medication with their patients and could provide them with information about the consequences of not following their recommendations, ultimately patients were at liberty to act as they wished. Rather than telling people what to do they considered they were providing information for patients to make their own decisions:

> Executive GP: I don't feel that I have to trust them to do what I say. Because that's not how I see myself as a doctor.
> *It does raise the issue of, well can you have confidence that they will be able to self-manage?*
> Yeah and I think it's er – I don't have a particular problem with

that, as long as I think that I've given them enough information that they understand it, that they understand the implications of their own decisions. So if they decide not to manage, for example, their diabetes, they understand that that means that they're going to risk complications that they could avoid.

Similarly, the diabetes nurse and the training GP suggested that with chronic conditions patients do have a real choice about whether to follow their clinician's recommendations and so they were not forced to trust patients to take their clinical advice.

Training GP: I think everyone has their own agenda for their own health care, or their own, you know, how they want to deal with things. And that's what I mean about, even if you decide that you're going to be prescriptive, 'You must do this,' they'll still turn around and rip up the prescription, or not get it.
Are you happy with that?
Um I think as long as people accept the responsibility that they take for their health care, yes. You know, that's up to them. Um it's frustrating, you know, and I mean it becomes more frustrating when you're talking about er a chronic disease.

The ambivalence that clinicians expressed in whether they could trust patients, as they were forced to in secondary care, or whether they needed to in the case of primary care contrasts with the patient perspective that mutual trust is important. Both diabetes and hip surgery patients were clear that they considered it important that their doctor or nurse trusted them as much as they trusted their doctor or nurse. This suggests that the 'patient partnership', described in policy discourses whereby patients work together with clinicians to address their health problems, is not being fully realized in current patient–clinician relationships.

DIMENSIONS OF TRUST

As previously described, trust is a multidimensional concept. On interviewing clinicians we found that across all occupations competence was a very important dimension of trust and that if clinical colleagues were incompetent then they would not be trusted. However, competence alone was not enough for trust between clinicians; other dimensions were necessary but they varied between primary and secondary care and across professions.

Competence

All clinicians talked about competence as being fundamental as to whether they would trust another clinician. However, what was meant by competence varied by clinical setting; a competent doctor in primary care could differ from a competent doctor in secondary care, as the executive partner in the practice explained:

> Executive GP: I think competence is very, very important in general practice, in medicine generally. Um but I think one of the key competences in general practice is being aware of the whole patient, and knowing what might be appropriate and what might be difficult because of the patient's circumstances, which I wouldn't necessarily expect a hospital clinician to know or be able to know.

Competence generally meant more than clinical ability and extended to include interpersonal skills.

> *So I mean, from what you're saying, you're suggesting that actually whether you trust someone or not is, to a certain extent, dependent on their competence?*
>
> Salaried GP: Yes I'd say almost entirely. I mean there's a sort of integrity trust, and then – but I suppose I'd put that under the umbrella of competence as well. So it may not just be clinical competence, it may be their competence to do the job when they're not in the mood or, you know, push through all of the barriers as well. It may be that they know all the causes of whatever it is [laughs] but not be good in their attitude, and I would count all of that ... And that may be knowledge about interpersonal skills as much as knowledge about big clinical stuff.

In the hip case studies all clinicians interviewed spoke of the importance of competence if they were to trust another clinician. For the consultants to delegate operating responsibilities to juniors trust in their competence was essential.

> Consultant: What you would do, you would limit clinical involvement initially until your confidence in them grows and you see them, they operate with you, you operate with them and you see patients with them. We have a hip meeting every Monday, they present cases, they are getting involved in decision-making. So you can hear how they are problem solving and if your confidence in them grows so they can do more and more over the period of time that they were with you.

Confidentiality, honesty, reliability and personal manner

For healthcare professionals reliability, honesty and personal manner were also important, that is competence alone or technical ability was not sufficient for trust.

> Diabetes nurse: And you know by their personality that they are the sort of person that would, um, they're conscientious, honest. You can think that somebody is competent to do a task, but if you felt that um the way that they were as a person they might do it in a rushed way or, then I wouldn't necessarily trust them. And I think a lot of it's got to do with honesty as well. I think um when I think of trust I sort of think of honesty.

> Fellow: Well I think with trust, I mean trust covers mainly – it covers that they are properly trained, well you sort of assess that, you know, they've got the skills levels. But that um – that also that they have common sense such that, say you're on holiday, and you've asked one of your colleagues who you trust to do – 'Can you look after these patients?' and something goes wrong with one of them. You see it's not just that they're reliable, but they've got the good clinical decisions and common sense to do that.

This was equally important for the nurses and therapists. According to one of the staff nurses, judging how competent nurses are depended not just on what you observed but also what they communicated to you. One of the occupational therapists said that problems arose when nurses did not trust other nurses to do things and had poor communication with one another as it created problems in handover with the therapists having to remind nurses what had to be done.

The doctors in primary and secondary care did not talk about confidentiality as being important for trust but it was important for all the nurses. The senior nurses thought confidentiality was important for their untrained staff and junior nurses to be able to trust them enough to talk to them about any problems. Similarly, for the healthcare assistants trust was needed if they were to confide in each other.

> Healthcare assistant: Yeah, there are people that you would speak to in confidence, and there are the other people that, no, you wouldn't do that. Um if I didn't trust them I wouldn't confide in them.

Confidentiality was particularly important for the ward receptionist who, because of her proximity to the ward leader's office, could hear many staff-related issues but could be trusted to not repeat them. In contrast, honesty was mentioned by many of the clinicians from all professions in secondary care as being important if they were to trust another clinician. In fact, lying was the main reason for clinicians losing trust in each other.

> Fellow: Um honesty I think is the most. You don't mind some-one not having done something, or someone having forgotten something, but if they lie, that's where I can't – that's where they get pulled aside.
>
> *What do you think trust means?*
> Ward Leader: I think it's about um – I think it's about honesty and reliability. And I think you know that that person is actually going to perform to a certain standard. They can – they would relay information accurately, they wouldn't embellish it, they wouldn't lie about it. Um I think that's probably what it means.

A dimension of trust that emerged in the hip case study but not diabetes was reliability. How care is provided within surgical teams, including the multidisciplinary input into patient care, made reliability key to clinicians' trust in one another.

> Healthcare assistant: You need to be able to trust somebody to be able to do the job, you know whether it's confidentiality or just to be able to rely on them to know that they're going to do what's required of them really.

For the doctors the new shift system introduced due to the shorter working hours required of doctors in training meant that reliability was even more important.

> Senior house officer: I think the foremost important is like: is he caring for the patient, does he spend time with the patients, and does he do what he says? I think that's it. Yeah reliability I think.

Reliability was important not only within a profession but between professions, for example for doctors to trust nurses.

> Staff nurse: Because at the end of the day, they come in and they say, 'We want this, this and this done,' well if you don't do it then they're not going to trust you to do it for them again. So, you know, you've got to be able to do your job competently. And you've got to be able to say to the doctor, 'Yes I've done that for

you,' or, 'No I haven't done this because of this, this and this.'
So there's got to be trust there.
Clinicians were divided as to the importance of personal manner.
For one of the GPs, personal manner and empathy were not import-
ant, although her personal disposition to trust others was relevant.

Some people would say, well actually personal manner is actually
what counts, that you end up trusting people just because of how
they are as an individual person.
Salaried GP: I don't trust people because I like them – I'm more
inclined to. I tend to trust most people when I meet them, in that
they give me no reason not to trust them. So my default would
be to trust them.

Another GP suggested that it was easier to trust people that you
liked and that for clinical relationships in this particular practice
both empathy and competence were necessary.

Training GP: I think if one comes down to pure trust, to some
extent, is it pure competence? Um and I suppose what I'm also
trying to think about a little bit is to do with empathy.
Yeah.
Um but I don't really think that that necessarily comes into
trust. I think it's easier to trust people with whom you have an
empathic relationship with. And there may be other doctors out
there who I don't get on with, but I still trust their clinical skill,
and that's a different.
If they are competent, but not empathetic, does it matter?
Depends on – I think, within this practice, it wouldn't work.

Acting in the interests of others

One way in which trust is defined is whether an individual acts in the
other's best interests. None of the junior staff in secondary care
referred to this but it was raised as being important for consultants
to be able to trust each other and other senior clinicians. At this stage
in their medical career there was scope for doctors to diversify in
terms of how much private practice they conducted, the extent to
which they were involved in research, and for different motivations
and interests to prevail. Competence in itself was not sufficient for
a consultant to trust another senior colleague; you might be technically very able but distrusted because you might not always act
completely in the patient's best interests.

Consultant: Competence, you could be technically competent and then I would not trust you, if you were not applying your technical competence for the right reasons . . . If you had somebody for example who was a bit flamboyant in perhaps how he treated his patients in the private sector, his indications of surgery were different there to the indications in the NHS. He can be a very competent surgeon but it would be difficult if you could not justify his motives it would be difficult to trust him.

In primary care clinicians did not refer directly to the need to be sure that their colleagues were acting in a patient's best interests as being important for trust, in part because this was taken as a given within the practice. The senior partner suggested an important criteria for selecting new partners had been whether they shared a similar motivation and value system. In her view the high trust between the GPs in the practice was in part due to the fact that they were all interested in research and training and in practising to the highest clinical standard, that is they shared similar motivations.

HOW TRUST IS BUILT AND LOST BETWEEN CLINICIANS

The creation of trust between clinicians and its loss depends on how clinicians define trust. In secondary care reliability, honesty and competence were the three key dimensions of trust identified by most clinicians; whether they trusted a colleague depended on the extent to which they displayed these qualities over time. Being honest about the limits of their clinical competence was particularly important from the nurse perspective, in generating the trust of senior nurses and doctors.

Ward leader: It's the trust that's grown over the years, and I know that they wouldn't willingly kind of do anything that would be detrimental to the patients, detrimental to the staff, detrimental to visitors. Um I know that if they came across a situation, or a procedure that they weren't familiar with, they would seek advice. You know, not everybody can know everything about everything. So it's the knowing that they know where to go for advice and help should they need it as well. And I'm very confident that they do.

Competence cannot be assumed in surgical teams due to the rotational method of training medical staff and the varying grades of nursing skills required for staffing a surgical ward. Competence had to be demonstrated and once senior doctors felt confident in a doctor's skills they would show greater trust in them by delegating greater patient management.

> Consultant: They come to you on a rotation so you have not selected them based on confidence. The clinical workload dictates that almost from the start they are going to have to be involved. It is not something you can protect the patient from the outset. You cannot do that scaled assessment at the outset. But what you would do, you would limit clinical involvement initially until your confidence in them grows and you see them, they operate with you, you operate with them and you see patients with them. We have a hip meeting every Monday, they present cases, they are getting involved in decision-making. So you can hear how they are problem solving and if your confidence in them grows so they can do more and more over the period of time that they were with you.

In primary care GPs assumed that their GP colleagues were competent although patients' reports and experiences provided evidence as to whether these assumptions were well founded. Trust between GPs and hospital doctors was built largely by communication.

> Salaried GP: Is there any trust? Yeah, I mean I think it's very difficult, partly not having trained in the area, that you don't feel that you have particularly strong bonds with them, you know. And it's – some consultants are very good at getting back to you and trying to sort things out for you.

GP trust in practice nurses grew with experience as they became more confident in the nurse's competence. As with doctors in secondary care, as GP trust in nurses increased and confidence in their competence grew then they would delegate greater patient management.

> Training partner: And so there is a possibility that she may take on the prescribing of those (diabetic treatments). Really, are you comfortable with that? I am with this particular nurse because I know the training that she's done, I've worked very closely with her on setting up an asthma clinic and in minor illness work and I know that she is um, that she would be a cautious prescriber, that she's not going to over-reach herself. And I know her background. Yeah. And I think if somebody else was going to start I would want to work more closely with them beforehand, that I would feel confident knowing their abilities.

Nurses also differentiated between the varying levels of competence that GPs showed in managing particular conditions. They recognised that GP skills differ and their trust in them to manage particular types of conditions varied accordingly.

> Diabetic nurse: Then there are other doctors who I don't know so well but their clinical judgement is absolutely spot on, clinically they are absolutely fantastic . . . And then there are others, you know, where you think well if I send this patient there that might not be the best doctor for them to see with that condition, because their expertise is somewhere else.

Many informants suggested that experience of working with a clinical colleague over time was necessary to create trust in their relationship.

> Consultant: No you can't, you can't, it's something that evolves. We can't come in together and say, 'Hello, I'm going to trust you if you're going to trust me.' When you've worked together for a while you build up trust.

But rather than time itself being important, it was the honesty, reliability and competence that clinicians displayed during a given period that was necessary in generating trust.

> *What builds your trust in another nurse?*
> Ward leader: Just, you know, from, one, looking at the patient, what their records are that have been written, what's been done, what needs to be done, what's handed over, their report, um what other members of the team say as well. You know, obviously I encourage teamwork, and if you're going to have someone that's not going to be part of the team, um people talk, people, you know, we all discuss.

> Registrar: I think in their attitude and their sort of behaviour and the way they approach things, then I think there's that, you know, you are encouraged to trust them when you see them acting at the same level of expectations as you have yourself.

The closer teamworking that was found within the surgical team, compared with primary care, also nurtured trust or distrust:

> Healthcare assistant: Friendship, um just working with people as a team, in a close team, doing lots of shifts together, I suppose you build your trust up like that really.

Trust between the nurses on the wards appeared to be particularly strong as they were very cohesive teams who had worked together over a long period of time. In contrast, junior doctors had less opportunity to build trust with the more senior doctors in the team due to their medical rotation. In fact, junior doctors had greater contact with the nurses on the ward and could develop closer trust relationships with them due to the frequency of their interactions.

Junior registrar: I don't have any problems trusting most of them. You know, I tend to find, because you work quite closely with the nurses, especially at this grade, you see them regularly, so you get to kind of make a judgement.

Finally, some of the nurses suggested that personality could contribute to building trust between clinicians in that an open communicative person could create trust more quickly.

What about time? Some people say you can build trust over time, do you think that's true?
Practice nurse: It is but I think you can accelerate trust. Yeah and I think that's through getting to know people better.
Right.
And it depends what sort of person you are as well really, your personality.
Right.
If you're quite an open person and you know, um quite chatty and communicate well, then I think you know, people get a better idea of what you are like.
Right.
Whereas if you're sort of a little bit more reserved, it takes people a longer while to establish what they think about you and trust you as well I think. So I think it does depend.

TRUST LOSING

In contrast to patients who found it difficult to talk about what might cause them to lose trust, clinicians easily identified key aspects of clinical performance which would cause a loss in trust, namely: clinical errors; being 'let down' by a colleague; and showing a lack of respect for one's peers.

In both primary and secondary care clinicians' trust in their colleagues depended again very much on the experience of their patients' care. If a clinician appeared to be underperforming or treating a patient inappropriately, either in terms of wrong medical care or because they were rude to the patient, then that would cause a loss of trust.

> *What would cause you to lose trust in a fellow clinician?*
> Executive GP: A fellow clinician, well um becoming aware that they were not – you know, underperforming, I suppose.
> *Like the GP?*
> Like the one that we had experience of, or if I had concerns about their mental health, or drinking too much, or whatever. Um I mean I think there were all sorts of clues in the other one, and reports from patients that they didn't think he would – you know, they weren't sure that he'd said the right thing or 'Why did he say that?' And, you know, sort of reports from patients saying, 'I didn't understand,' or patients saying that someone was rude to them, or didn't listen to them, that kind of thing.

Patient complaints per se would not necessarily reduce their trust in a clinical colleague; it would depend on the nature of the complaint and whether the problem arose a number of times. Similarly, in the surgical teams' errors and poor patient care would cause clinical colleagues to lose trust in each other if it occurred on a number of occasions.

> Staff nurse: If I felt that they weren't doing their job to the best of their ability, and it wasn't a one-off occasion. This is like over, you know, months, you know, if I notice that their work is starting to slide, they're not as reliable, they're not communicating, they're not – you know, and I'm thinking well, you know, I'd chat to them to see if we can resolve it. And – but yeah, if their work was sliding, sliding down, and nothing we were doing was helping them to get back to where they were.

So, just as trust takes time to be built up so trust is lost over a period of time, although probably a briefer period, due to problems like treatment not happening when it was supposed to.

Clinical errors may not lead to a loss of trust but they will do if they cause a colleague to feel 'let down' in some way. This was particularly the case in the hospital setting where clinicians are so reliant on multidisciplinary input into patient care. Doctors, nurses and therapists suggested that if a clinician failed to do something they had been asked to do or failed to turn up to meetings or proved unreliable in some other way, they would lose trust in them.

Occupational therapist: I mean certain people that we liaise with, especially sort of external to the hospital, we trust to start off with that they're actually going to be doing that, but um from past experience when things – we've been let down and things haven't happened when a service is supposed to be provided. An external service is supposed to be provided by a certain time, or we're told it's going to be a certain time, and it doesn't happen, um so then you don't actually trust that.

Similarly, all professions suggested that if a clinician was not honest then they would not be able to trust them.

Registrar: I think if you then establish later on that someone hadn't told you the truth, I think if you'd been lied to that would be about the hardest thing to then forgive. Because no matter what you say at that point you're going to be thinking, 'Well are you lying to me again?'

Some of the nurses and therapists also reported that if a colleague failed to keep some information confidential then they would lose trust in them.

Staff nurse: And also if I um – if I was talking to them and I said, 'Look, this is between us, alright, not to go outside.' And then the following week I got back and everyone was, 'Oh you've told so and so this,' and I'm thinking, 'Hang on a minute, that was supposed to be in confidence,' I'd lose trust in them, and I wouldn't tell them any kind of maybe confidential information again.

Clinicians might also lose trust in each other if they failed to show adequate respect for them as 'clinical colleagues' and in particular if they failed to respond to requests for information.

Practice nurse: I think it would be something really like if I could never access them, if I could never get hold of them, if I kept leaving messages and they never replied. That sort of thing, I think I would just think, 'Well I'm not going to bother any more.'

It is interesting that none of the clinicians suggested that performance data would influence the extent to which they trusted a clinical colleague. Personal characteristics such as honesty, reliability and confidentiality, as well as a clinician's technical and communication skills, built and lost trust between clinicians rather than information collected for performance monitoring or clinical governance purposes.

Clinicians' loss of trust in patients depended on the nature of the consultation and what they were trusting them to do. A practice nurse might feel uncomfortable about seeing a particular person alone due to concerns that they might be violent or aggressive and they would seek a chaperone in such circumstances. Clinicians might lose trust in patients with long-term conditions and their ability to manage their condition if the patient either did not seem to understand their illness or dismissed it lightly. If they did not trust the patient to self-manage, this would lead to more active management by the clinician. In secondary care many of the doctors had little trust in patients' willingness to follow their rehabilitation advice after discharge because they had seen patients ignoring their instructions when out in the community and because they had to manage those who returned to hospital after dislocating their hip.

One of the consultants said that they were more likely to specify in detail in writing if they did not trust the patient and thought they might make a complaint.

> Consultant: I think when you're aware that somebody's maybe upset or a bit more challenging, and you think that maybe they're going to um complain, or just put it forward a bit more at a later point in time, you will be more aware of writing down real specifics.

HIGH TRUST AND LOW TRUST BEHAVIOUR

The level of trust between clinical colleagues was expressed in three main ways: the extent to which patient care was delegated and monitored; the type of communication between clinicians; and the extent to which they supported each other in their clinical tasks. Specific behaviour which indicates high and low trust is detailed in Table 4.1.

Trust within professions was evident in the extent that senior nurses, doctors or therapists felt able to delegate clinical tasks to their junior staff. This was particularly important for GPs who shared patient lists.

> Salaried GP: I think people are confident about delegating and then just letting stuff go, which presumably implies there's either lack of care or significant trust, and I'd hope it was the latter . . .

Table 4.1 High and low trust behaviour as identified by clinicians

High trust behaviour	Described by clinicians	Low trust behaviour
Limited supervision and checking that work has been done	X	Constant monitoring and increased supervision
Delegation of patient management	X	Limit clinical involvement
Significant professional autonomy	X	Little delegation of authority
Not anxious about holiday cover	X	Concerned by cover
Praise patient management	X	Criticize patient management
Seek advice from a particular clinician	X	Avoid asking advice from a particular clinician
Accept clinical opinion	X	Seek another clinical opinion
Openly seek help with a task that is beyond your clinical competence	X	Do not voice concerns about your competence to do a given task or seek support
Raise concerns directly and informally with a colleague or discuss first with peers	X	Speak to senior clinician about concerns regarding a colleague or use formal complaints procedure
Good communication, informal and unwritten	X	Poor communication, often formal and written
Good teamworking	X	Poor teamworking

I mentioned delegation earlier – I think you would find it very hard to delegate to somebody you didn't trust, you'd feel you retained that responsibility for whatever it was.

The diabetes nurse reported that her limited supervision and ability to delegate tasks to the other nurses and healthcare assistants were important signs of trust.

Diabetes nurse: Um but it's very hard for me to sort of actually specifically be there and supervise, you know, so there is a lot of trust involved. And I have to, because otherwise I would just be [laughs] going demented.

This was confirmed by the healthcare assistant who suggested that the limited monitoring enabled her to act on her own initiative. Among the GPs monitoring was similarly limited, even supervision of trainee GPs was described as 'hands-off'.

> Salaried GP: I had a slot in the week where I could go to her if I wanted, but I didn't have to, and I went less and less. And I also had an appraisal sort of three times a year with her, as a retainer.
> *Right.*
> But in fact, I was a retainer for such a short period of time I had one. And it was useful, but I mean that was all it was. Um so yes, I mean it wasn't particularly hands-on supervision, no.

The GP responsible for training said that in-house clinical appraisals were not necessary because their work was regularly observed for training purposes. Although the practice appeared to have a high trust culture with very limited clinical monitoring, the receptionist said that occasionally the GPs did check up on each other to ensure that something had happened when worried about a particular issue.

> Receptionist: It has happened in the past and, you know, you think – you know. And they're continuously saying to you, 'Did Dr. So and So do this today? Did he do that visit?' Or – as though they're checking up on that doctor. And then, to me, I start thinking, 'Hmm what are they thinking?' They're obviously a little bit worried about what's happening.

In secondary care, limited supervision and an ability to delegate to junior staff grades were essential to effective teamworking and a sign of trust within professional groups, for example between occupational therapists or between doctors, and between different professions.

> Registrar: And he [the consultant] looks at the cases very much: the straightforward primary cases, those are for me to do under his supervision, you know, being taught to become more slick really, in terms of how I carry out the procedures. And the more complex revision cases are for the senior fellow to do, so he's ready in six months or a year's time to be an independent consultant.

Limited checking that work had been completed as requested and to an appropriate standard was evident of trust between clinicians irrespective of their professional background.

And what about say between a nurse and a doctor, what would you trust them to do?
Ward leader: I would take that as being you trust them to do the care that is required of them as a doctor, um adequately enough without us having to check up on it really.

Ward leader: Well I suppose you don't have to check up on everything all the time, and you feel that you don't have to um do that because you know someone else is going to do it. You know, you know that your B Grades will write the care plans, will do the obs, you know that they will come and tell you if there's anything that they're worried about. You don't have to go and check every single temperature, whether they've got one, because you know that they are reported to you. So it just makes for more of an efficiently run ward, I feel.

One of the physiotherapists also confirmed that checking on work done – by one of the other members of the multidisciplinary team – would be an indication of low trust.

Physiotherapist: I think, if they didn't trust me, they'd be spending half their time complaining [laughs] about me, or um checking up on the work that I'm doing really. I think if they didn't trust me from a multidisciplinary point of view, I think I'd know pretty quickly.

When there was less trust in a clinician's competence and colleagues expressed concern that a clinician was struggling or having problems, then the difficulty was discussed and monitoring and supervision was increased.

Confidence in another clinician's management of patients was another way in which clinicians showed their level of trust in colleagues. If doctors trusted their colleagues they were not anxious about them providing cover while on holiday or if they worked part time in managing their patients on the days that they were not in the practice or hospital. The executive GP suggested that when they trusted their hospital colleagues they would not worry about checking how patients who they referred were managed; they were confident that the problem would be sorted out and that they would have come to the right decision about their management.

Executive GP: If you can refer to someone that you have confidence in, that you do trust, then you can feel that you won't have to check up on what happened when the patient went there, that it will have been sorted out and that, you know, they'll have been helped to come to the right decision about their management.

Criticism of clinical colleagues signalled low trust. If a GP had low trust in a hospital doctor they might criticize their management of patients and avoid referring to them again if possible.

Executive GP: If you refer to somebody that you don't trust, then you will be more likely to have the patient coming back saying they don't understand, they were being told they had to do something they don't want to do, or have an operation they don't want to have. Or you might, you know, and this particularly happens I guess in terms of admissions, that patients come out and you find that they've not been sorted out at all, and that's distressing and very, very dangerous really.

Similarly, in the closer working environment of secondary care, criticism of a clinician could easily create and spread distrust within the team. One of the junior doctors gave an example of how criticism of another clinical colleague could spread distrust among colleagues and patients even if this was unwarranted:

Junior registrar: And the problem is, if someone then turns round, and I did this once, I overheard one of the nursing staff slagging off someone, and I had a go at them, and I said, you know, 'You shouldn't say that,' and they were like, 'Why not?' I said, 'Because you don't know that for a fact do you?' And the reason I said that is because I knew the facts. And I said, 'You don't know that for a fact.' And she was like, 'No.' I said, 'That's alright, I know you're an alright person and you're just saying it because you're stressed. But the problem is, is there's five other people in the room who've heard you say that. Now if they have a different interaction with that person that's adverse again, the first thing they're going to do is remember your conversation, and they will lump together and make out that he's crap. And that's not true.' And that is what goes on. And patients overhear this.

Low trust might result in criticism but before reaching that stage it could make clinicians wary of accepting the clinical opinion offered by a colleague. Nurses might voice wariness of some of the junior doctors if they did not appear to be learning on the ward and if they were wary of one of their clinical colleagues, they would seek someone else's opinion as well. For senior staff low trust might manifest itself in terms of suspicion regarding what was motivating their peers towards a particular course of action. Such suspicions might result in consultants failing to agree a common course of action.

> Consultant: People will be fairly outspoken but if you actually wanted to, would we agree that this is the way that we are going to go forward and it actually means action, so are we going to withdraw a service unless somebody does something? But that very rarely happens and there is this: 'I would look at you wondering what are you trying to get out of this, and you are thinking I wonder what he is up to now.' I am not sure that that is trust, there is quite a lot of suspicion of the motivators of why your colleagues are doing what they are doing. And of course there is also this private practice thing.

The other way in which clinicians showed the extent to which they trusted one another was in the nature of their communication. When there was high trust between clinicians this was reflected in the informality of communication methods between staff. When one of the consultants was away from the hospital he would call to check with the ward leader on the recovery of his patients.

> Ward leader: Um, you know, he [the consultant] rings me up from wherever he is in the world, and we do the ward round over the telephone, and he trusts that I will give him accurate information. He will ring me up and say, 'What do my X-rays look like?' And I'll say, 'Well this one is so and so, and that one is so and so.' You know, 'And what are the wounds like?' Yes I know what all the wounds are like, because I'm very involved in the care.

Similarly, the nurses would telephone the ward leader at home if there were problems with any of the patients.

> Ward leader: So any issues they would sometimes ring me from home and say, 'Oh by the way, this has occurred.' And any problems, you know, with theatres or relatives or, you know, there's a whole load of things that could crop up they would keep me informed. They may well have dealt with it, but they will say, 'Oh by the way, this happened, you know, if anyone says anything to you about so and so, this is what it was about,' and so we communicate in that way really.

High trust promoted good communication and staff could be open with each other. One of the staff nurses suggested that if she had concerns about another nurse she would raise her concerns directly with them first and talk to them informally or ask her ward leader to have an informal chat rather than going through a formal written complaints procedure. Similarly, junior and untrained nurses were willing to say if they did not feel competent to do something whereas in a low trust environment it would be harder to be so open about your possible 'shortcomings' as they might be used against you.

> Staff nurse: The HCAs we have on the ward here are very good. I mean if they felt they weren't competent to do something they would actually say, 'I can't do that job, R, I'm sorry.'

Good communication assisted teamworking and high trust promoted more effective delivery of care. In a high trust environment staff reported being more ready to support each other and help each other if part of the team was busier than others, whereas in low trust teams communication was poor and clinicians were less open with each other about their views regarding how a patient was being managed, even if they had concerns.

> Fellow: I've worked in units where nothing was – you know, certain members of the department never spoke to each other because they didn't get on. And then it would be extremely difficult, because one would never be able to discuss with the other and say, 'Well I don't think you should be doing that,' because they just couldn't.

Both nurses and doctors talked about targeting requests for advice or support. They were careful to seek advice from specific doctors who they could trust to help with a particular issue, avoiding others who they did not trust.

> Salaried GP: I target who I ask certain things from, but er – and I suppose that, in terms of trust, there are some doctors who I know have weak areas on some issues, and I wouldn't trust them with that topic, but they wouldn't trust themselves either, so that's fine [laughs] you know, they know they are their weak areas.

Low and high trust were also demonstrated by the different ways that concerns about the competence of a clinical colleague were handled. Where there was high trust between colleagues, doctors or nurses would speak to each other and check out their concerns first before raising the issue with their fellow clinician.

If you lose trust in a clinical colleague, what do you do about it?
Training partner: Yeah um I think um someone like within the practice, probably I would make sure it wasn't me first. I know that sounds odd but. But I think, you know – you know, I'd probably have a word with one of my other partners to begin with and say, 'Look, you know, I think something's a bit odd here – is it me, or have you had any issues as well?'

Only after speaking informally to their colleague would they raise it with a more senior member of staff.

Registrar: If you say, 'Look, you know, this happened, I came to talk to you about it and, you know, what you told me wasn't true. So why? You know, why have you lied to me, you know, what's going on? Is there something else going on that's, you know, affecting the way you're acting? Or is there a reason why you did that?' And I think at that point you say, 'Look, should we have a chat with, you know, one of the registrars or, you know, one of the other SHOs?' You know, eventually, if you carry on following that process you're going to be involving the doctor's consultant. And I think, if what they've done is very serious, then you're left with very little choice but to do something like that. But I'd never do that directly without sort of going and talking to the person and saying, 'Look, you know, this is serious.'

The occupational therapists and physiotherapists took a similar approach, going back to a person if there was a concern, and only then speaking with their manager. In extreme circumstances where a clinician actively distrusted the clinical competence of their peers or seniors, then they might take the ultimate step of changing jobs. One of the nurses talked about how her lack of trust in her clinical colleagues in a previous job had caused her to seek new employment because she did not consider it to be clinically safe.

BENEFITS AND DISADVANTAGES OF TRUST

The benefits of trust between clinicians brought advantages not just for the individuals involved and their working relationships, but for the organization they worked for. Some of the doctors in both primary and secondary care considered trust essential to effective working relationships.

> *Is it important they [other GPs] trust you?*
> Yes.
> *If they didn't trust you, why would that be a problem?*
> I think if they didn't trust me then I would feel that the relationship would break down.

One of the consultants suggested that it was fundamental for the surgical team and the system of surgery to function well. If a colleague was away then the consultant would help out and vice versa. Trust appeared to promote better working relationships by encouraging openness and good communication and fostering respect.

> *If you're trying to unpick the specific value of trust to an organization, what would you say that it brings to it?*
> Practice nurse: Ooh I think it would be the hinge pin on the smooth running of an organization really, trust. If you haven't got trust then things don't work well generally . . . Um, you know, communicating in itself, you probably wouldn't – if you didn't trust somebody you wouldn't be so eager to communicate with them, so you may not gain their support in management of patients so well.

> Physiotherapist: Um because I think if you can gain somebody's trust, you educate them more effectively. Um if they trust you, they'll listen to you more, and then follow advice more readily, I think. I think if they don't trust you, you're not going to build up a rapport. And not necessarily that they're not going to take the information onboard, but it just doesn't make for good working relationships really.

Trust helped to build respect between clinical colleagues and between patients and clinicians and clinicians and managers, which is discussed in Chapter 5.

One of the organizational benefits of trust was that it appeared to make services more efficient because there was less checking and clinicians were able to delegate tasks.

> Occupational therapist: Um I think you can work more effectively together when you're trusting the other person. Um it also is more time efficient, because you don't have to double-check up on things. And that you can take one word, you haven't got

to get it double-checked with someone else. Um so I think, yeah, I think it makes closer working relationships.

One of the ward leaders saw mutual trust between clinicians as being important for an efficient ward as well as being good for patients. Several of the other therapists suggested that by promoting more effective teamworking, trust was essential for good clinical care and for good relationships with patients.

Occupational therapist: Yeah just it just affects the whole team dynamics, doesn't it, if you can't trust your – your team, then er the whole clinical er patient's experience falls – falls down.

Although clinicians recognized that trust made for better relationships with patients, encouraging better concordance with treatment and appropriate use of medication, they did not identify it as contributing to better health outcomes.

Practice nurse: And also you need to be able to trust from a medication point of view, if you're asking them to take certain medications, you have to trust that they're going to be able to take that appropriately, and not have any mistakes or mishaps, especially where diabetics are concerned.

In the hip case studies clinicians also suggested that trust was important for patient concordance with recommendations regarding post-operative rehabilitation.

Senior house officer: I trust most of them. I think so, because if I ask them to – if I ask them to do this thing, and if they do that, like even mobilizing or anything like that, if they don't do that and then I won't be – I won't be that pleased or happy. Because it's my trust in them that if I operate upon them, like if my boss operates upon them he trusts them to work hard after that.

Other organizational benefits that clinicians identified included: people taking less sick leave, less office politics, more effective use of clinical time because of low DNA rates, good teamworking and better staff retention.

Salaried GP: I think it's incredibly difficult to work as a team with people you don't trust . . . Um I think it would lead to a very stressful working environment, which obviously has problems all the way down the line.

The only disadvantage of trust identified by clinicians was that you might be let down by colleagues that you had trusted too much and mistakes might have been made because you had either over-delegated to or under-supervised someone.

And are there any disadvantages if you trust your colleagues?
Salaried GP: I think if you trust them inappropriately, yes. I think you can um – I think you can over-delegate, and you can under-question. Um so I think mistakes can be made because you presume greater knowledge than is there.

Consultant: Well if you're going to take junior staff, and they're going to do something for the first time, or early on in their training, you are going to take a knock with your results, let's be quite clear about this. If you look at the [situation of] arthroplasties, for example, registrars have ten times the dislocation rate of a consultant.

In the acute setting nurses talked about being let down not due to clinical incompetence but because another nurse might have failed to retain a confidence. When this happened and there was a breakdown in trust between nurses, then it created problems and inefficiencies because they would not help each other out.

Receptionist: If they, you know, have their little disagreements or, you know, they're not talking to each other, then, you know, nothing will get done. Because the other person will say, 'Oh I'm not going round to help out, she's working that side, because I don't talk to her. She can go, you know, and work orange, and I won't go and help her.' You know, there is no teamwork there, there is no – there is nothing.

The doctors in secondary care identified problems in trusting someone to do something for their patient, it not happening, and the patient having problems as a result.

Senior house officer: Yes like if I am away on leave, and I leave some um – I ask somebody to care about those patients, and if they don't care about them, or if there is any problem. And obviously with the orthopaedic hips and knees they are mostly elderly, so even if you don't check them for two or three days, like you don't see them quite often, or don't get there, like if they are long term here, I think they get – they tend to get infections and things with the hospital.

One of the occupational therapists suggested that if there was too much trust, you might not be cautious enough and things might get missed because you were too relaxed.

Occupational therapist: If it's all trusting and then there's not that cautious side to it, then things might get missed. Because if you're not chasing things up then, yeah, from experience, you do need to kind of keep re-evaluating things. And um although I sort of trust them that the intention is there, the job might not get done, therefore it needs to be reviewed.

One of the staff nurses also suggested that patients might not voice their concerns quickly enough if they had too much trust in the clinical team because they would think the professionals always knew best. If a patient appeared to trust one nurse to do particular things more than the other nurses then this could create bad feeling. In general, however, there was a clear sense that trust brought with it many benefits and that the potential disadvantages of trusting too much were minor.

CONCLUSIONS

When discussing trust with clinicians in the two case studies, it became evident that trust between health professionals was very important, both between colleagues in the same discipline and between different disciplines. In primary care the nurses interviewed considered that it was important that they trusted the GPs to provide clinical support and for the GPs to trust the nurses.

Is it important that you trust the GPs, and the GPs trust you?
Practice nurse: Oh yeah it's imperative really. And hopefully they do. I think, you know, you have to be confident, but also um you have to know your own abilities and be cautious. So confident with caution, I think that's really, from the nursing point of view, what the GPs are looking for.

The system of delegating within medical and nursing teams and relying on other professions to provide their input into patient care meant that trust was essential to effective patient care.

Do you think trust is important, that clinicians trust each other?
Practice nurse: Yes I think so, yeah very important. You have to.

First off you have to trust their abilities. That's probably where I would have my biggest problem, is trusting people's ability to do something. And if you're – if you're – obviously you're not going to see a patient, if I work one end of the week I might not see them at the other end of the week if it's dressings or something like that, and you have to trust your colleague to be able to look after them as well as you, perhaps not the same as you because you're not the same. So I mean yes, trust is important.

When asked whether trust was relevant to their relationships with patients, clinicians considered it was important for patients to trust them but were less sure as to whether they needed to trust patients.

It appears from the case studies that the importance of trust and its increasing salience is in part due to changes in the way that healthcare is organized and delivered. The loss of personal GP lists, the increasing involvement of nurses and other health professions in clinical decision-making and patient management, and the use of new working hours and medical shift systems in secondary care have increased health professionals' reliance upon each other and made trust between them important for effective working relationships. Trust relations also appear to be affected by differing clinical contexts; the close teamworking in secondary care surgical teams enables clinicians to directly assess whether an individual is sufficiently honest, reliable and competent to warrant trust, whereas in primary care clinicians use more indirect information such as patient reports to determine whether they can trust a colleague.

However, there were many similarities between clinicians and their understanding of trust, irrespective of the clinical or organizational setting. There was agreement that competence was a key dimension of trust but that other dimensions, notably reliability and honesty, and in particular an awareness of the limits of their clinical competence, were necessary. Trust was conditional in that it had to be earned although the altruism of other clinicians was generally assumed, except at the consultant level. As with patients, performance data appeared to have no influence on the extent of trust between clinicians; rather trust was earned through clinical interactions and communication which acted as opportunities to demonstrate competence, honesty and reliability.

Clinicians did show some differences in their attitudes to trust. For nurses, confidentiality was more important, perhaps in secondary care because of their greater or more intimate patient contact. Junior clinicians, both doctors, nurses and therapists, felt it was important that they showed caution and demonstrated that they were aware of their clinical competencies in order to win the trust of more senior clinicians. Likewise, among the HCAs in primary care and the junior doctors in secondary care, there were still signs that traditional trust relations persisted whereby senior staff were trusted simply due to their seniority and place in the medical hierarchy. However, with this exception, clinician to clinician trust does reflect our proposition that trust needs to be mutual and is now conditional and has to be earned. As with patients, there was some evidence of forced trust in secondary care where clinicians had to trust the new shift system to work and they were forced to trust that patients would follow their rehabilitation advice following discharge. It was evident from interviews with clinicians how trust could be constructed and lost, and they talked much more readily than patients about low trust and distrust in some of their relationships with clinicians, patients and managers. It is these relationships with managers that we now explore.

5

TRUST RELATIONS BETWEEN CLINICIANS, MANAGERS AND PATIENTS

In previous chapters we have discussed the role of trust in relationships between patients and clinicians and between healthcare practitioners, drawing on previously published studies and a theoretical framework to suggest how these relations might operate within the UK NHS. In this chapter we examine the nature of trust in relationships between managers and clinicians in the NHS, and to a lesser extent between managers and patients. We draw solely on the findings of our empirical work into trust as no other published research has investigated this particular relationship. In so doing we are mindful that our conclusions must be cautious in that this exploratory study can only suggest how these relationships may be operating. Further research is required to explore trust relationships between clinicians and managers and between senior and middle health service managers in other organizational settings.

THE NATURE OF TRUST RELATIONS WITH MANAGERS IN PRIMARY CARE

In primary care clinicians and patients may come into contact with managers at two different organizational levels: the practice manager at the surgery and managers employed by primary care trusts (PCTs), and NHS organizations which have a responsibility for commissioning care for their local population and managing and providing community services. One of the major developments within general practice in the last decade has been the changing role of the practice manager. GPs have always required assistance with the administrative aspect of running their surgeries and traditionally this was a very limited role, often undertaken by former receptionists or informally by partners. With the growth in size of practices and the more complex mechanisms for securing payment for services, practice managers now need financial, human resources, information technology (IT) and administrative skills and experience to be able to manage these small businesses. The practice manager in case study 1 fitted this new mould of practice manager. He had considerable experience of management outside the NHS and had been recruited by the GPs for the generic skills that he could bring to managing the surgery. The practice manager, clinicians, and to a much lesser extent patients, may come in contact with managers at the local PCT. In our primary care case study we interviewed the PCT manager with responsibility for managing general practice development and who was one of the key managers that GPs liaised with at the PCT. A pharmacist by background, this manager had been working with practices in the area for a number of years and was well placed to describe relations between GPs and the PCT.

In the theoretical framework in Chapter 2, we suggested that traditionally clinicians and managers had an unequal relationship whereby managers were expected to trust clinicians because of their professional status, and the ethos, expertise and autonomy that came with it. As managers essentially performed a supportive administrative function, there was limited need for clinicians to trust managers. In the 'new NHS' clerical staff continue to provide administrative support to clinical staff, but a manager's role extends to advising on and at times determining how health services are to be organized and delivered. In this more equal relationship, managers have been given greater influence due to their budget-holding responsibilities and through initiatives introduced by central government including clinical governance and performance targets. Clinical governance requires clinicians to demonstrate to senior managers within their organization, or in general practice to the PCT, that they are meeting clinical standards and improving the quality of care. Performance targets such as limiting waits in Accident & Emergency to four hours enable managers to identify where services need to be improved and to instigate change in how services are provided in order to increase their efficiency and ensure that their organization does not incur financial penalties for failing to meet a target. The new responsibilities of NHS managers and their enhanced role led us to suggest that trust relations between clinicians and managers would now need to be more mutual and that trust would need to be earned based on the performance of both clinicians and managers.

In primary care clinicians did talk about the need for mutual trust between themselves and both the practice manager and PCT managers (see Figure 5.1). Clinicians within the practice agreed on the importance of being able to trust the practice manager. For him and the clinicians within the practice trust needed to be mutual, the manager needed to trust the GPs were being honest with him and the rest of the staff while from the GPs' perspective trust was earned by a manager's competence and ability to solve problems.

Practice manager: As I say, that's the reason why I probably get a lot of time to do what I do is because they trust my decisions, my experience, um and they've seen the rewards of that. Just be managing certain areas, you know, they've been rewarded, either through, you know platitudes or through remuneration.

Executive partner: I think that doctors did have a problem in thinking that they knew how to do everything and that managers were a nuisance and jumped up and should damn well be quiet and do what they were told. I think that has changed and I think that doctors now trust and respect managers more than they did. Even if they don't like what they're doing.

Is that true for secondary care?
Possibly less so, because it's so much bigger and less personal but it's certainly true of general practice.
Practice manager: As I say, I trust them to give the people around here the sort of clinical skills that they require . . . if I

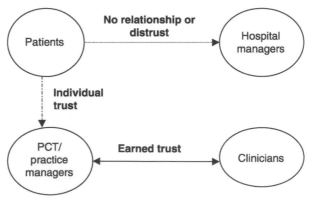

Figure 5.1   Trust relations between clinicians, managers and diabetic patients

didn't trust them then the relationship wouldn't continue. I can't work in a situation where I don't trust my superiors to either upset the customer or upset the staff that we work with. You know, my prior job to this I probably moved because of that issue, that we'd get told one thing and we' d be not quite sure if that's exactly what's going to happen.

The PCT manager also talked about how trust between the PCT and the practices was conditional and that it needed to be earned through relationships with the practice managers and GPs. For some of the clinicians within the practice who had no contact with the PCT, they neither trusted nor distrusted managers because they had no relationship with them. The practice manager and clinicians who had contact with the PCT considered that trust was necessary for an effective working relationship and that it was earned in part by managers being honest with clinicians and them delivering on their promises.

Diabetes nurse: I have to say when we have practice nurse meetings at the PCT that the PCT nurses has [sic] always been, you know, very open and honest about what's going on at the PCT ... You know they are trying to let us know about things.

The PCT manager held quite an instrumental perspective on the need for trust, suggesting that trust is important only when you need GPs' cooperation to do things differently.

PCT manager: I think if you're trying to get people to do things differently then you do need them to [trust you]. But if you're just buying the same old thing that you've always bought, you don't really care ... We need to keep them working with us rather than against us. And um I think respect, trust and mutual understanding, all those things are important.

Patients had no comments to make on trust in primary care managers as they had no relationship with them; instead, when asked about trust in NHS managers, they exclusively referred to their distrust of hospital managers. Half the diabetes patients interviewed considered that there were too many managers and that they distrusted them because of reports and experience of dirty hospital wards and poor food.

Diabetes patient: Given local managers have failed in basic simple things like hygiene and food – they are not rocket science

– and they can't even get them right – so I don't think I can trust them.

Do you trust people who manage the NHS?
Patient 2: No, its obvious isn't it? The hospitals aren't clean. I don't mind paying money in, but I don't like the fact that it's paying managers money, paying for a manager doing silly things like um cutting down on the food that they have.

The other diabetes patients expressed similar concerns that there were too many managers but reported that they could either probably trust managers or at least did not actively distrust them. Although both the PCT manager and the practice manager recognized that they had limited dealings with patients, they considered it very important that patients could trust them in individual interactions and sought to build patient trust in them. They recognized, however, that managers generally would always be made the scapegoat for problems within the NHS and hence distrusted. They did not consider this a problem as long as it did not impinge on their job.

PCT manager: I think that where we do have direct contact with patients, most of my interventions with patients are pretty positive. If they've written with a complaint or they've written with information, I think by and large our experience is positive.

Practice manager: I don't think it's a problem if patients don't trust management. I think it's going to happen anyway. It's different for a manager here, it's a much smaller environment and it has to be that they trust what I say and get the issue resolved for them. In a faceless hospital I don't think it matters, they're always going to have some scapegoat and the managers are going to be the ones that they choose over the doctors and nurses.

The developing role of health service managers has changed the clinician–manager relationship and at least in some parts of primary care it now reflects one of mutual trust and respect.

THE NATURE OF TRUST RELATIONS WITH MANAGERS IN SECONDARY CARE

In secondary care patients and clinicians may come into contact with three different types of manager in addition to staff such a.

receptionists and medical secretaries who provide administrative support. Clinical managers are clinicians who have largely dropped their clinical workload to take on a managerial role; in this case study we interviewed the nurse manager who was responsible for all nursing staff on the orthopaedic wards. Directorate managers operate as middle managers in hospitals; they have responsibility for the effective delivery of services within their directorate, including the meeting of any targets set by senior managers, and hold the budget for the directorate. Directorate managers report to senior managers, the executive team who are responsible for the overall running of the hospital. In the secondary care case study we interviewed the manager responsible for managing the orthopaedic directorate but were not able to interview any senior managers.

Figure 5.2 illustrates the various trust relations between clinicians and patients and these different types of manager. In this case study clinicians had better relationships with clinical managers enjoying mutual trust; the managers were respected for their clinical background and clinicians considered that the managers had more empathy for the difficulties they faced in providing services.

> Nurse director: In my case I've worked up from a staff nurse to a sister to a matron, and I think I quite like that, because I've been there, I've worked on the wards, OK not for a few years now, and you can understand where the issues are and sort of empathize.

Trust was conditional between them and was earned through competence and a manager's accessibility. Nurses of all grades could access and have a trust relationship with their nursing manager, whereas only senior clinicians directly interacted with the directorate manager, although other staff were able to comment on this relationship. The senior clinicians who we interviewed did not have a management role within the organization, other than their responsibility for junior medical staff. Without access to the managerial perspective on problems facing the service, they tended to distrust the directorate and senior managers who they considered had differing agendas to clinicians and whose competence and honesty they doubted.

> Registrar: 'I think there's been a lot of tension for years when – since um there's been sort of non-medical managerial staff trying to um, trying to run services based on targets and performance and numbers, rather than clinical need and priority.'

It was evident that senior clinicians were frustrated with having to

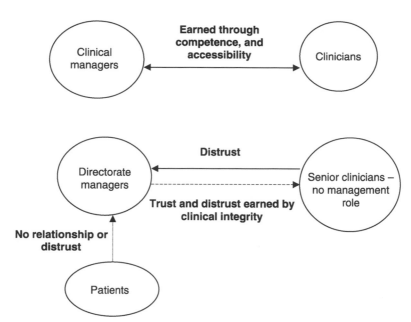

Figure 5.2 Trust relations between hospital clinicians, patients and managers

negotiate with managers for resources and to accommodate targets which impinged on their clinical autonomy and how they would like to run services. From the directorate manager's perspective, whether they trusted or distrusted a clinician depended on their clinical integrity, whether they put patients' interests first. The directorate manager felt squeezed from all sides because as well as being distrusted by some of the clinicians, she also talked about not being trusted by their senior managers who were often unavailable and unsupportive to this middle tier of personnel and to the clinicians. The manager recognized this distrust.

> Directorate manager: There's definitely an us and them sort of thing . . . I think the trust's senior management team, um, what the doctors say is they're not visible enough, they don't hear from the horse's mouth often enough what really is happening.

Similarly, patients, if they made a comment on their trust in managers, tended to voice distrust of them due to problems with hygiene.

> *Do you think people who manage the NHS can be trusted?*
> Hip patient: No, because it's so obvious isn't it, the hospitals

aren't clean? People are dying and some of them are, some of them die because the hospitals aren't clean.

Although there was evidence of mutual respect and trust between clinical managers and clinicians, the relationship between clinicians and directorate managers was typically one of distrust. The different types of trust shown in primary and secondary care and the reasons for the lack of trust in clinician–manager relations will now be examined and evidence for how trust could be rebuilt explored.

TYPES OF TRUST

In the theoretical framework in Chapter 2, we suggested that trust relations may have changed from a one-sided relationship when the professional autonomy and power of clinicians did not require them to trust managers to a situation today when there is a need for greater mutual trust because managers are reliant on clinicians to achieve their performance targets and clinicians are reliant on managers to secure the resources they would like. When individuals are dependent on each other, there is an opportunity for trust to develop if each party seeks to cultivate the trust of the other. We proposed that we might find a shift from status trust, where managers were forced to trust clinicians due to their professional status, to a performance-based trust where clinicians and managers would earn each other's trust by delivering what the other needed.

On interviewing the executive partner of the case study practice, it was evident that she had witnessed this change in the clinician–manager relationship.

> Executive GP: I think that managers used to be very distant people that didn't have much to do with clinicians. Um and I think that they've crossed the boundary. Yes I think the managers have become much more hands-on. And I think initially that was resented, and particularly by consultants.
> *In determining how services are run?*
> Yes, yes. In the old days when I was a junior doctor, the consultant was the boss of the service. And, you know, what he wanted to happen happened. And that's not the way it is any more. The managers manage the budgets and I think that interface has changed. And I think that that means that it wouldn't work if relationships weren't good enough.

Do you think trust comes into that?
Yeah I think it does, I think that doctors did have a problem in thinking that they knew how to do everything, and that managers were a nuisance and jumped up, and should damn well be quiet and do what they were told. I think that that has changed, and I think that doctors now trust and respect managers more than they did. Even if they don't like what they're doing.

CONDITIONAL AND UNCONDITIONAL TRUST

According to most of the clinicians and all the managers interviewed, trust was conditional in that it had to be earned. The only exception to this was one of the GPs in the practice who had little contact with managers at the PCT but assumed she could trust them. She assumed that she could trust managers' decisions, on the basis that they have the information to hand to make the right resource allocation decisions. She trusted that decisions to cut services were made by people who knew the bigger picture far better than she could and she also recognized that it would be very demanding on her resources if she did not trust managers.

The other GPs in the practice suggested that trust was earned over time and depended on the effectiveness and honesty of managers. A number of secondary care clinicians also suggested that the honesty of managers was important in earning their trust but they also needed to show an understanding of clinical concerns. For the nurses this understanding of clinical issues could be earned by managers being more accessible, coming on to the ward and seeing how things are done.

> Staff nurse: I think there's probably always the thought of 'them and us' yeah. Because they're not on the ground. I think ward staff would say, 'I wish they'd come here and just see what it's like.' Because they don't. And so there is always that feeling of, 'Oh why are they saying this?' They haven't got a clue.

From the manager's perspective, the PCT manager suggested that trust between managers and clinicians could not necessarily be assumed and that it had to be earned.

> *The other thing is, do you have to bother to make, to build up trust, or can you just take it for granted?*
> PCT manager: Um I don't think you can take it for granted. I

think a lot depends on what you've done before. And I think you might be able to take it for granted initially, but I think once you've lost trust, you know, you can't assume you're going to have it next time.

Both he and the practice manager talked in terms of performance trust; whether clinicians trusted them depended on their competence and delivering what they said they would do.

In the hip case study managers also talked about performance trust in that they considered that clinicians could earn their trust by whether they are helpful to managers when they had a problem, whether they were honest, and by how good they were with patients.

Directorate manager: And I do get – I get a lot of feedback from the various different professions, the nurses in the clinic, and waiting list coordinators, and the physiotherapists, about how people [medics] treat patients. So I think primarily it would be on their reputation, and how they get on with, how they are deemed to treat patients, and whether they are fair. It's also whether I think they are fair in their dealings with us. I mean some doctors are um – are very er helpful in terms of sorting out, particularly waiting list problems. Um and others are not very helpful in doing that, and they're unnecessarily obstructive sometimes.

One relationship which we did not explore in our empirical study but which was touched on in some of the interviews was trust between managers. In secondary care the directorate manager talked about 'forced trust' and how they had to trust that other managers would tackle a problem they had presented them with.

Directorate manager: Well because I rely on them providing services to allow me to function in this job, you know. So the medical records example, I mean I have to trust my general manager that manages the medical records side of things, that he will do his best to provide me with a good medical records service. And um, you know, I need to know that he recognizes that I've got a problem.

DIMENSIONS OF TRUST

Competence

When investigating trust between clinicians, and between patients and clinicians, competence emerged as the key dimension of trust. In contrast, when exploring trust between clinicians and managers, competence only appeared important in primary care whereas in secondary care other dimensions such as honesty and working in each other's interests emerged as being more critical to trust. This is not to say that clinicians in secondary care would trust an incompetent manager; rather that there were other dimensions of trust which had greater influence on trust before competence was considered.

In primary care competence was important for both clinicians and managers to establish mutual trust.

Practice manager: I would trust that the clinicians are treating the patients favourably, that they're actually administering them correctly, that they're maintaining their status and their learning to current thinking. I trust them to give the people round here the sort of clinical skills they require.

Does competence come in, is that a big issue?
PCT manager: I'm sure it must be, yeah, I'm sure it must be. And as I say, it's like I said before, it's about you delivering what you say you're going to do, you know, implementing change properly. Um I mean, for example, with the QOF, I mean it was a new system to implement, we needed to devise data collection methods, devise a system of practice visits, run those meetings sensibly, and I think my impression is that – I could be wrong – but my impression is that actually we did that reasonably well, and that the practices felt we did it – in fact I think we got a letter from the practice manager saying they thought it was a good job.

In secondary care the manager claimed that she could not judge a clinician's clinical competence, although she went on to explain that they did get feedback about a clinician's clinical skills so they were aware of which clinicians are good.

Honesty and accessibility

In the hip case study, honesty, integrity, accessibility and reliability were more significant attributes of trust between clinicians and managers. Managers trusted clinicians if they considered they were honest and acted with integrity, for example whether she believed holiday booking forms or whether she could trust doctors to be in clinic when they said they were.

Directorate manager: Well I think if people are honest about the way that they deal with things. Um whether people are um – you know, always turn up for their clinics, always are there when they should be at the end of their clinics. And their own consultancy should be in clinic from this period to this period, and quite often if you pop down there, they're not there, and then you have to wonder where they are.

Nurse manager: Um honesty at all times really. If a mistake is made, being up-front and us sort of learning from the experience. Um a credible practitioner.

Honesty was also important for clinicians if they were to be able to trust managers.

Consultant: I think I would be much more confident about what I do in my job if I could go and speak to the managers, which one does, if you have a problem you go and see one of the senior managers. If I could go and speak to them and say this is what I want to do, these are my problems and they gave you an answer, and the answer may not be a correct answer but if they were giving their answer in true honesty . . . From my point I am absolutely sure they are profoundly devious.

When talking about managers that were trusted the consultants explained why.

Consultant: I think he was doing a good job, I trusted him, I thought that if I went to him for something and it was just not on the cards he would come right out and said you have not got a hope in hell of it.

For the nurse manager being accessible was important and also an indicator that she was trusted because nurses would come and confide their problems in her.

Nurse manager: Well I hope they do. Um I think, you know, I do have a sort of steady stream of nurses coming to see me about various things, so I think if they didn't, you know, I'd catch up [laughs] with my paperwork.

This was confirmed by one of the occupational therapists who recounted a bad experience of a manager who had not been very professional and so she had avoided her.

Occupational therapist: Well we had some problems with a manager who was um quite unprofessional, . . . and the issue um being bullying really. Um and um so no, I didn't trust her to um deal with things effectively and professionally. And to be honest, in the end I ended up – you just wanted to avoid her, because anything that – it would just turn sour.

Acting in the Interests of Others

The other key dimension that was important for trust between clinicians and managers but not for trust between patients and clinicians was whether clinicians felt managers were acting in their interests or working to a completely different agenda. One of the GPs considered not just competence but the extent to which managers acted in the interests of the practice as important as to whether they trusted them. The fact that the PCT had to follow the government's agenda meant the GP could not necessarily trust them.

> Executive GP: Um I trust their integrity, I don't think they're, you know, awful people or dishonest or crooks or anything. But I think they have an agenda that's different from ours. Um which is driven from the government, and target-led. Um and that's mixed with a desire to do the job and do the best thing for patients. And they find themselves in big conflict with the PCT. *Right, right.*
> Which means that we can't trust them [laughs] very far.

For the hip case study clinicians this was the fundamental reason for why they had such low trust in managers. Consultants' lack of trust that managers were acting in patients' best interests caused them to distrust them.

> *Do you trust managers?*
> Consultant: Not an inch.
> *Why not?*
> Because they're solely interested in advancing themselves up the greasy pole of management, and satisfying central directives from government which are inappropriately targeted.

> Consultant: The previous manager X . . . because we trusted him he was removed. I thought he was doing a really good job, but he was just a little bit too friendly with the consultants. He was too sympathetic for our concerns.

The directorate manager recognized that it was important that she was honest in her dealings with clinicians if they were to trust her but this did not remove the fact that she was working to a different agenda.

> Directorate manager: Um I think they need to be able to trust that you're going to work with them, and that you're not going to – as a manager I think you need to make sure that you're not sort of trying to go behind their backs. Because if they don't trust you on that, then if you wanted them to do something for you, at the end of the day they're just not going to do it, are they?

HOW TRUST IS BUILT AND LOST BETWEEN CLINICIANS, PATIENTS AND MANAGERS

The ways in which trust can be built and lost depend on how it is defined; thus, for managers' relationships with clinicians, honesty, accessibility and competence were key to trust construction. Managers also suggested that 'being reasonable' was another mechanism whereby they tried to nurture trust.

Managers in both primary and secondary care sought to build trust in them by 'being reasonable'. This may reflect that managers are aware that historically relations between clinicians and managers have been adversarial and that this was something they need to overcome.

> *How do you think you build that trust?*
> Practice manager: Um, that's mainly just by being fair, I think. You know, I've not always agreed with what they want, but if I give a fair reason why I don't they respect it . . . And so here it's like 'Yes that sounds good but we can't do that because of this reason.' And I think they trust my fairness to do these things I do.

> *So what builds trust between you?*
> PCT manager: Um, I think it's quite often simple things, you know. If you say you're going to do something, do you do it? Um, do you make stupid suggestions? You know, are you reasonable, do you act reasonably? It's not about always doing what they like but I think a lot of it is about being reasonable and acting in a reasonable manner.

Similarly, in secondary care providing clinicians with a reason for change was important in encouraging trust.

> Directorate manager: If you've got things that you want to change, or you want to introduce, or are being sort of devolved

from on high, that you can come and you can explain it, and you can tell them why it needs to happen. And I think most of them are quite amenable if you've got a good explanation of the benefits of it.

Managers also reported competence as being important, although they expressed it in managerial terminology stating that trust is earned through delivery or proving themselves.

PCT manager: It's like I said before, it's about delivering what you say you're going to do, you know, implementing change properly. In the previous section we already identified that honesty was particularly important for clinicians in secondary care to trust managers.

Consultant: We used to have one manager here, she was great, a girl called X. She worked late at night, dead straight, dead fair, and everyone trusted her.

Face-to-face contact was also important in building clinicians' trust in managers.

Practice nurse: To be honest, he's very proactive, X the manager here. Right. He's very proactive, you know and he sees you. Very different from the last practice manager. Right, just because he sees you? Yeah.

Accessibility was similarly important for clinicians in hospitals to trust managers and if managers had been more visible out on the wards it would have increased trust still further.

Nurse manager: No, I try to maintain a sort of policy where I'm accessible and visible at all times, I carry a radio page, um I've got an open door policy, and so if staff need to speak to me I'm available for them, or if they want me to go down to the ward.

HCA: If you don't see the manager, if she was in the office all the time, you'd feel perhaps she didn't care or – do you know?

Clinical managers benefited not only from increased credibility with clinicians because of their clinical background; they were also well known to clinicians from when they were working on the wards. As a result the nurse manager was able to develop more informal relations with clinicians and she recognized the importance of being accessible in encouraging them to trust her.

Ward leader: Um a lot of them know Z from her being a sister anyway, and a lot of them may well have worked with her. Um so a lot of them will just go to Z, um or ring her up, or see her in the corridor and, you know, talk things through there.

When patients talked about their trust in NHS managers, their remarks referred solely to hospital managers; those that work in primary care are essentially invisible to them. For patients cleanliness was the key mechanism whereby managers could build trust in them and their hospital, with cleanliness being seen by some informants as a symbol of the hospital's efficiency and managerial competence.

What would a hospital have to do to encourage you to trust it?
Diabetes patient: I'd have to see the efficiency and the cleanliness. In fact you can tell a good hospital by the cleanliness of the place. Right. What does cleanliness say about an organization? Efficient . . . It will bounce off all the way through, you get a clean ward, you get a happy ward, you get an efficient ward, the treatment goes well, the patients feel better.

Performance data in the form of star ratings or league tables were not regarded as being effective in building trust with patients in either case study. When they were mentioned patients dismissed them as being manipulated.

What about when you hear how well a hospital is doing in the league table?
Hip patient: Well I know [laughs] I know how they fiddle the numbers you know. We're both adults, aren't we? And we know it is just a fiddle.

TRUST LOSING

Clinicians' trust in managers appeared to be closely aligned to whether they had shared interests; where their agendas diverged trust was easily lost. In both primary and secondary care clinicians said that they would lose trust in managers if they appeared to be making meeting government targets a priority over clinical need.

Salaried GP: And I think, you know, no one likes being told what to do, and managers putting their foot down. And I think particularly if you've got an ignorant manager who is managing purely on numbers with no recognition of what you're trying to do essentially, and no recognition of the human component of medicine, then that's deeply, deeply frustrating, and can very much limit what you're able to do.

Physiotherapist: I do think working on the ground, grass-roots level, um I suppose often we take a bit of umbrage maybe with certain managers, or maybe as it goes higher up the ladder. Because I know that they have financial targets to meet, and er I can appreciate that, but at the end of the day I have to make sure my patients are safe.

Consultant: Clearly there are managers in the hospital who impose guidelines on what we are meant to be doing. I think living by political intervention they will impose goals that are not in accordance with the clinical priorities that we identify.

The directorate manager recognized the conflict in terms of prioritizing operating lists in order to meet her targets and to meet clinical need:

Directorate manager: Because, you know, they just don't – the consultants want to list people in what they see as clinical urgency, and we say, 'Well, you know, this patient has been on the waiting list six months, therefore that makes them urgent now, you know, you have to treat them.' And then if they've got a patient that they saw last week that they think has a more clinical need than the patient who has been on the waiting list for six months with their () or whatever, it's a dilemma to, you know, to do both.

She considered waiting times and central targets as having been very destructive of trust between clinicians and managers. However, one of the clinicians suggested that targets per se did not necessarily have to be divisive, it was the manner in which managers interacted with clinicians that caused problems and in part their accessibility, visibility and approach.

Fellow: Yeah, because they're not – I mean I think amongst clinicians, you know, there's this perception of there's this terrible divide. And you work in some places where managers do get involved, and it makes the place so much better. But in a lot of places you're not, you're just sent, you know, 'Can you make sure you don't cancel the fourth case on the list today?' and that's the only input you'll ever get from the management, apart from telling you off. Yeah well in our speciality, at present, that is the case. It's not how it was previously. Previously we had people who we would speak to on the corridor and, well we'd speak to them, you know. But our directive – I hate the phrase – line managers in that respect, at present are very much 'send directives' which often are contrary, to us clinicians, our perception of what is the best treatment for the patient.

Fellow: You see a lot of what's gone on in the NHS for many years was, 'Look, we're running a bit late, but can we go on a bit longer to get this patient done?' And the answer has invariably been yes, OK. Now it's being thrown at us, 'Get this patient done.' It's relying on the goodwill that has always been there in the NHS to meet their targets. 'Get it done. You'd better not cancel this,' OK. Once you start treating people like that, you're no longer treating them as – you know … But if managers manage by coming down and being part of the team, as they did previously, you really feel that you've done it for everyone. Whereas now, as I said, as we discussed at the beginning I don't feel loyal to the managers because they don't treat us with respect necessarily.

Another reason for why clinicians in secondary care distrusted managers in the hospital was that their involvement in running the service was seen as interference with clinical decision-making and indicated a lack of respect for clinicians' professional judgement and autonomy. Distrust was created particularly when clinicians felt managers were interfering to save money but this resulted in poorer patient care:

Fellow: And (managers) saying to the nurses, 'Use this product.' If the nurses say, 'This causes more blisters on the skin, we don't want to do it,' OK, 'Use it, it's 20p cheaper an item.' That's – you've taken their professionalism away, you're not interested in their opinion any more. And the same is happening with the doctors etc.

Senior house officer: So I don't think so. I wouldn't trust them if they start meddling into things, 'This patient should get this because this implant is cheaper,' or, 'he should get this medication because this is cheaper,' I don't think so I would trust them then, because then they are not bothered about, or interested in what – what the primary job is, to take care of the patients. You know, managers are normally there to smooth everything, it's not to just put blocks and things in the working of NHS.

In primary care there has been considerable change in the organization and structure of PCTs and with that has come changes in personnel. Where trust in managers was based on knowledge of a particular individual and their particular management style, then constant change of personnel made it harder for clinicians to trust managers.

> Practice nurse: There's a big impact that comes from the PCT, and I think because things almost seem to be changing by the minute, I think that's really quite hard, I think, for the doctors and nurses to trust and to know, 'Well what's going on, sort of thing, who do I talk to? How do I get the right information?' I think that can be quite hard.

With regard to their relationship with patients, managers felt that negative media coverage was in part responsible for their lack of trust and they were very critical of what they regarded as being irresponsible coverage.

> *What about when you hear criticisms of the NHS generally then, when people are saying, 'Oh it's all down to the managers'?*
> Practice manager: Well unfortunately that's the media, and I – I – since I've taken this job on, I've stopped reading the papers. Yeah, because I've seen – because it's a bigger political football than I think I ever used to work in. And I never gave it too much notice, you know, I'd read the paper and go, 'Oh bloody hell, look what they've done in the NHS.' And now that you're actually in amongst it – and I mean the flu thing, I think that's the one that capped it for me, when they said like, you know, 'Oh there's going to be this big flu epidemic, etc., etc.,' and everybody flocked in and had a flu injection. And then the following week they were saying, 'Doctors scare patients, and there's flu vaccine shortages.' And you go, 'Hold on, you did that last week.' And I think that was the cap, and I went, 'That's it, I don't read a paper from now on.'

They also suggested that patients' limited contact with managers did not encourage patient trust in them. Patients did frequently comment that there were too many managers and this was probably stimulated by media reports, but it was their personal experience either directly or indirectly via friends and family of the cleanliness of hospitals and the food provided that affected their level of trust in NHS managers. In fact, when patients did complain managers saw it as an opportunity to restore trust or confidence in the service.

PCT manager: I don't think they do have very much contact with managers. And I think that where patients – where we do have direct contact with patients, most of my interventions with patients are usually pretty positive. If they've written with a complaint, or they've written for information, I think by and large our experience is positive. And similarly when we have laypeople involved in PCT work, either – they're not really laypeople – but non-executive directors, you know, we have user groups, patient forums, I think the relationship is pretty good. I think we do tend to get a bad press. I think that er we tend to get quite a lot of, you know, the reason why the Health Service has overspent is because it's bad management, and sometimes that's true.

When managers were asked what would cause them to lose trust in clinicians, they suggested that dishonesty and lack of integrity were the prime reasons for a loss in trust. The only reference to performance was made by the nursing manager who said that she would lose trust in a nurse if she made drug errors.

HIGH AND LOW TRUST BEHAVIOUR

The extent of trust between managers and clinicians was reflected in both the nature of clinician–manager communication and the way in which managers monitored clinical activity. There was a strong contrast between the two case studies in the extent of trust between clinicians and managers. In the general practice case study both clinicians and the practice manager talked about the high level of trust in their relationship which had been nurtured over two years since the practice manager had come into post. The practice's GPs also seemed to have a reasonably good relationship with the PCT. In contrast, in secondary care clinicians voiced low trust and in some instances distrust of the hospital's middle and senior managers. Trust relations only appeared to be good between the nursing staff and the director of nursing.

The differences in levels of trust between clinicians and managers in the two case studies was reflected in the high and low trust behaviour that respondents identified and which is summarized in Table 5.1. The extent of checking, monitoring and supervision was a key indicator

Table 5.1   High and low trust behaviour as identified by managers

High trust behaviour	Described by managers	Low trust behaviour
Light touch monitoring	X	Detailed checking that work has been done
Share confidential information	X	No discussion of confidential information with managers
Accept at face value people's motives	X	Express suspicions about a manager's or clinician's motives
Readily access managers	X	Avoid managers
Good communication, informal and unwritten	X	Poor communication, often formal and written
Good teamworking	X	Poor teamworking

of how much managers trusted clinicians and vice versa. Within the PCT the practice manager was given considerable autonomy in how he organized his work and in decision-making and the GPs generally relied on him and sought him out when they required their assistance rather than closely supervising him. The PCT manager also identified limited monitoring as a sign of trust between the PCT and practices. He cited the way the PCT monitored the implementation of the Quality and Outcomes Framework as an example, stating that such a light touch was necessary for GPs to buy into the contract.

> *The data they provide, you trust is accurate, rather than you constantly going in to check?*
> PCT manager: Yes so, you know, the QOF standards say you get 15 points if you've controlled these patients' blood pressure, you know, we don't go out and recheck blood pressures, we don't write to patients and say, 'Are you actually being prescribed these drugs that the doctor has been saying you are?' So it is a high trust environment.

In contrast, over an issue where the PCT had less trust in the practices, the manager was prepared to undertake much more detailed monitoring to check on how money has been spent.

> PCT manager: We're about to do a piece of work um on how some money that was given to practices for PMS growth has been used, where the additional money was given to practices as part

of particularly the PMS contract for delivering certain other objectives. And the deal was that the money was going to be used for doctors and nurses, that's what it had to be used on. And so we are going to go back to those practices now and say, 'Well right, please give us the names of people that you employed with this money, and the dates for which you employed them.' So that's maybe a slightly lower trust, in that we're not happy that we've just given them the money and they've gone away and spent it as they said they would. We're going to go back and get the details.

It is of note that the PCT manager was going to check on whether the money had been used to employ staff, not on the extra clinical activity or quality of care provided, indicating the limits to which they can check clinical behaviour in general practice.

Another way in which clinicians in primary care showed their trust, not just of the practice manager but of the administrative staff in general, was their willingness to discuss confidential information in front of them and share patient information with them.

> Receptionist: I think probably it's more open today. Um I mean doctors will talk about patients in front of us. I mean I've gone up to the common room when they've been discussing a patient, but obviously our confidentiality, it goes no further, and they know that. But I've never, when Dr. X was here, she would never discuss a patient in front of a receptionist. That's how it's changed, in that respect.
> *Do you think that's a good thing or a bad thing?*
> I think it's good, because going back to trust, they obviously trust us that, confidentiality, we're not going to take it any further. And they know obviously by us working with them for so long, they know probably that they can trust us. Um and sometimes it does help, because if I pick up on something they've said, and maybe that patient rang, and I've thought, 'Oh they're discussing her, they must want to speak to her,' and I can follow it through in that respect. So I think to keep us informed and communicate on something. Whereas that, in Dr. X's day, we wouldn't have known that was going on.

Expressing suspicions

In both primary and secondary care, if clinicians distrusted a manager or vice versa this would be reflected in suspicions they voiced about each other's motives. The executive GP, when talking of her trust in the practice manager, said that although generally she trusted people by default, not trusting somebody equated to being suspicious of them.

> Executive GP: I'm probably fairly trusting in trusting him (practice manager) to be sure really [laughs] I have complete um – you know, I would usually give people the benefit of the doubt until I had good reasons to be suspicious of somebody.

One of the receptionists who did not have such high trust in the practice manager did express suspicions of his motives and whether if she went to him with a problem, whether she could trust that he would act in her best interests or resolve the problem effectively. In such circumstances she would go and speak to one of the GPs.

In the surgical directorate several clinicians expressed cynicism about the manager's motives, suggesting that her only concern was climbing the management ladder and therefore she was not motivated by patient concerns. In a similar vein the directorate manager indicated her low trust of some of the consultants by expressing scepticism regarding their productivity:

> Directorate manager: And when you look at their productivity, you sort of do have to question whether they're being as productive as they can within their normal working hours, um and whether they're just making more of a problem of their waiting list, and then reaping the benefits because we have to pay them to do extra work. So there is an issue for me about, you know, whether I think people work hard, whether I think that they um – that they're fair with their patients.

Where clinicians and managers distrusted one another, they were more likely to put things in writing.

> Directorate manager: And so I'll always be covering my back with those people, and I might follow things up more in writing, I might um talk to my clinical director about certain issues with them that, if the same thing happened with another consultant I possibly wouldn't, because I trust them that they're – you know, their motives of doing things.

It was evident from comments made by a variety of clinicians in the surgical team that the directorate manager was not considered part of the team, suggesting that their distrust of each other hampered teamworking. One of the therapists talked about how they actively avoided certain managers because they were considered obstructive and unhelpful. In contrast, the nursing director had developed good relations with the nurses and they were happy to go and find her and discuss any problems with her informally. This suggests the extent to which managers are involved in clinical issues and clinicians' willingness to seek them out to discuss problems reflect their trust in a manager.

BENEFITS AND DISADVANTAGES OF TRUST

Managers suggested that trust brought benefits to them as individuals in their relationships with clinicians and to the organizations they work in. The practice manager proposed that trust promoted more efficient use of clinical time by encouraging GPs to delegate clinical tasks to the nurses and healthcare assistants, as well as other organizational benefits including better staff retention.

> Practice manager: I think that relationship between the clinicians and the nurses is one of trust. And I mean to the point where we are training our nurses up to actually do things like minor illness clinics and things like that, and take on more responsibility for other things.
> *And the clinicians are comfortable with that?*
> Yeah, yeah because they see it as, if we can do that end and deal with – we're always looking at – if I say if we look at the lowest denominator for things that can be done, you know, so an admin person should be doing admin, not a doctor, if a nurse can be doing emergency surgery whilst the doctor can do complicated um routine appointments with their patients that they don't get to see that often. You know, so you're always looking for who can do that job, which is the person that can do it?

The practice manager also suggested that GPs have reaped financial rewards by trusting his decisions.

> Practice manager: Because they trust my decisions, they trust my experience, um and they've seen the rewards of that. Just by managing certain areas, you know, they've been rewarded, either through, you know, platitudes or through um remuneration.

Both the practice manager and the PCT manager identified trust as being key to effective working relations with practices. PCT manager: 'Because, you know, we make promises, we do deals, and

I think if they can't trust us then um it makes relationships very difficult.' He also suggested that it contributed to management efficiency as it cuts down on monitoring of activity and verification of payment claims.

> PCT manager: I think you've got to have some trust, otherwise your management costs would be completely spiralling, because you'd have to have all these people doing post verification of so much.

In secondary care the nurses suggested that a key benefit of being able to trust their nursing manager was that they could seek her help in solving problems. Trust encouraged junior nurses to talk to her if they had a problem with their line manager.

> Staff nurse: You've got to be able to trust your managers. Because if – you know, if they've got um an issue on the ward which hasn't been dealt with, with the ward manager, and you need to go to your managers, or if there's like um – there's just something which you can't talk to your managers, you can always go to somebody else. That is quite important, you know, that you have a good relationship with them, and that you are able to trust them.

Senior nurses also felt able to confide their problems and they recognized that trust meant they were not overly supervised.

> Ward nurse: Even if you just want to go and have a whinge and a moan, you know it won't go any further, you know she respects you in what you do as a manager, um she's not on your back all the time, she trusts what you do, and the decisions that you make, um so yeah.

The nursing manager in secondary care did not identify any disadvantages; in fact, from her perspective without trust you could not progress anything.

As would be expected in a situation of low trust, the senior clinicians in secondary care could not identify any benefits of trusting the directorate manager. Instead, they talked about the disadvantages of being let down by managers who had promised extra resources and then failed to secure them:

> Consultant: We have been let down on so many occasions, even now that we speak. Some of the circumstances are beyond the managers' immediate control. If I ask can we get five thousand

pounds and you say the reason I asked you to get that is so we can do some serious research, these are the problems but let's see if we can put this in and see if we can initiate this, and we might get the money. Don't say to me we have got the money and then I start planning that we are going to get the money and we can't get the money. There is not that sort of transparency.

Like the clinicians the managers suggested that the disadvantage of trusting too much is that you might be let down. When this occurred the repercussions identified by managers were that it might compromise patient safety and it might be a waste of public funds.

What's the downside to trust?
PCT manager: Um I suppose the downside is that you can get led astray, you know, you can get let down. And, you know, the risk there is that you're risking the public purse and wasting money, as well as putting patients at risk because they're not getting the levels of care that they need. So there's certainly a downside to trust, yeah.

CONCLUSIONS

Despite the greater extent of trust between clinicians and managers in primary care compared with colleagues in secondary care, informants in both cases acknowledged the importance of trust and considered it fundamental to effective working relations between clinicians and managers. The practice manager considered it particularly important that the GPs in the practice trusted him as he was managing their funds. He also considered it important that there was mutual trust between the practice and the PCT to ensure an effective working relationship. For the PCT manager trust was important as it reduced management monitoring costs as well as making for effective relationships.

Do you think trust is important?
PCT manager: Yeah, I mean I think otherwise you would – I think you've got to have some trust, otherwise your management costs would be completely spiralling, because you'd have to have all these people doing post-verification of so much. And it's just getting that balance right. And I guess, you know, you'd just get some real difficulty for practices to actually deliver a service if there's no trust there.

Do you think it's important that they trust you?
I think it is important that they trust us, yeah.

The managers in secondary care considered clinician–manager trust as being important if they were to progress anything but they also recognized that there were low levels of trust.

Directorate manager: I think it's important that you know who you trust.
Is that new?
I think it's always been important.
Why?
I think it's important, but I'm not sure they do trust us. I mean some doctors are um – are very er helpful in terms of sorting out, particularly waiting list problems. Um and others are not very helpful in doing that, and they're unnecessarily obstructive sometimes.

Some of the distrust expressed by clinicians in managers in secondary care may reflect frustration and resentment that some clinicians may have felt about the change in power and influence in clinician–manager relations and their need to work with managers in delivering services. However, clinician–manager distrust cannot simply be ascribed to professional resentment due to a reduction in their clinical autonomy. The same consultants who voiced distrust of senior and middle managers also talked about managers who they had trusted. Clinicians' trust in managers was conditional but it could be earned by a managers' approach – their accessibility, visibility, honesty and competence. Clinical managers, like the director of nursing, seemed to intrinsically recognize this and as a result enjoyed much better trust relationships with colleagues.

Most importantly, unlike other trust relations that we have explored which identified competence as the fundamental building block of trust, acting in the interests of others or rather the sense that clinicians and managers shared (or did not share) interests and a common agenda was the key dimension of trust. Where clinicians considered that managers were operating to a different agenda, primarily dictated by government targets which might conflict with clinical need, trust was lost. To a certain extent managers acknowledged this and recognized that if they were 'reasonable' and delivered on promises, then they could build clinicians' trust in them but from our research such effective working relations were only being achieved in primary care not in our secondary care case study.

Changes in the management of primary care with the development of the practice manager role and the introduction of greater, if still limited, accountability to PCTs have changed the nature of trust relations as proposed in our theoretical framework. In our primary care case study trust between clinicians and managers was mutual and depended on performance, that is competence and delivery, but it is likely that the same might not be found in other practices where the practice manager may not have such an independent role or in other PCTs where managers may not have sought to engage GPs as much. Similarly, in other secondary care settings we might find less distrust between clinicians and managers because managers may have taken a different approach, seeking to engage clinicians and encourage joint ownership of the targets services have to meet and trying to align them with clinical needs.

It is evident from this research that the type and frequency of interactions between clinicians and managers has a strong influence on the extent of trust between them. Where there is no interaction, such as between some GPs and the PCT, or between patients and managers, then there may be neither trust nor distrust, they simply do not have a relationship. However, for some patients direct interaction was not necessary for them to decide whether they trusted hospital managers; they used their experience of hospital visits as a proxy indicator of management competence and efficiency. Where hygiene standards were poor, patients interpreted this as a sign of managerial incompetence and hence they distrusted them. Managers to a certain extent dismissed such views as being generated by the media but it was clear from our interviews that patients were quite cynical about media coverage and they based their opinion on their own experiences. Is it problematic if patients distrust managers? Some of the managers suggested it was not if it didn't affect their job, but this fails to consider the wider implications for hospitals, both in terms of attracting patients if they are distrusted, and for the wider NHS if NHS hospital managers appear incompetent at running services. How much longer will the public continue to support a health service which they do not trust to be able to achieve basic standards of hygiene? These wider implications of trust and distrust between clinicians, patients and managers will be examined in our concluding chapter.

TRUST STILL MATTERS IN HEALTHCARE?

The overall aim of this book was to examine the nature of trust relations in the NHS. The focus throughout has been on the need to explore the different levels and types of trust relations that constitute interpersonal, organizational and institutional trust In the earlier chapters we presented a theoretical framework based primarily on an analysis of the policy and sociological literature depicting how trust relations may have changed. The explanatory power of this framework and the concepts embraced in it were explored empirically by examining the salience and nature of trust relations in different clinical and organizational contexts in the NHS. In this concluding chapter we begin by assessing the findings of our research into trust in healthcare relationships within the UK NHS, between clinicians, managers and patients. We then examine the implications of these findings for theory and for policy and for institutional trust in the NHS as a health system. Finally, we identify a number of thematic areas which might be explored in future research based on the evidence from our and others' research.

TRUST FROM THE PATIENT'S PERSPECTIVE

Our research into patients' trust in clinicians and managers suggests that trust is still very relevant to their relationships with individual practitioners. Patient trust in clinicians can no longer be assumed; it is increasingly conditional and has to be earned. However, it is important to recognize that there are still some patients who prefer to have blind trust or assume trust in doctors and nurses simply due to their professional status, authority and expertise. This appears to resonate with other research which suggests that in some contexts patients prefer a more passive stance whereas in others they are more active and even consumerist (Lupton 1994; Stevenson and Scambler 2005). Alternatively, it might reflect the social position of the informants who participated in the study who were drawn from the older age groups. Evidence from research into patient satisfaction shows that the most consistent pattern of relationships between satisfaction and indices of social position is for age, that is satisfaction levels with healthcare increase with age, and the relationship is a linear one with the most marked increases occurring in people in the 50–60 year age group. There is a range of explanations for this but whether this pattern is also evident in the case of trust remains to be seen (Allsop 2006). However, even if this linear and positive relationship between levels of trust and ageing holds up, it might have been expected that the use of blind and assumed trust would have been more prevalent among this group of informants.

Clinicians can earn patients' trust through their competence, their ability to communicate as well as their technical skills, and the empathy they show. Patients do not use information to judge whether trust is warranted; instead, they base their trust on their experience of care. If patients have a positive experience of care, then their trust in a particular practitioner will grow but if it is negative then such trust will fall. As a result, every healthcare encounter could act as an opportunity for the growth or decline in trust. The centrality of the patient experience to trust generation is illustrated in Figure 6.1 This illustrates that the effects of a good patient experience increases not just patient trust in clinicians and managers but also in organizations.

Increasingly, patients want trust to be two-way, considering that it is important for clinicians to trust them as much as for them to trust healthcare professionals. Mutual trust is important not just for patients with a long-term condition. Patients undergoing elective hip surgery considered mutual trust equally important but for them trust was sometimes earned and sometimes forced due to the complexity and acuteness of their condition. This suggests that for patients who do not have any elective component to their care, trust will be very important but it may be entirely forced rather than earned. From the clinical perspective, practitioners were more ambivalent about whether it was important for them to trust patients. For patients with long-term conditions clinicians felt that it was up to the individual whether they followed their advice and that they as GPs or nurses did not have to trust them. In contrast, in secondary

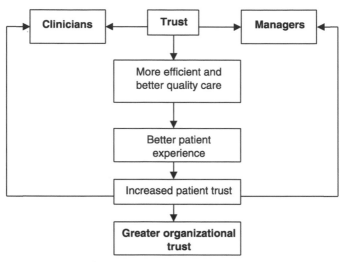

Figure 6.1   Reframing trust relationships: trust creation

care the surgical team felt they were forced to trust patients to follow their advice about rehabilitation post-discharge. Their dependence on patient concordance was higher because if patients did not follow their advice, they would be back in hospital with a dislocated hip.

Greater patient participation has changed how clinicians interact with patients both in terms of the information they provide, the amount of respect that they show them and how much they involve them in decisions regarding their treatment and care. If a clinician did not trust a patient to manage their long-term condition they would see them more frequently. However, we found only one instance when a patient's trust in a clinician was dependent on the information they provided and whether they could answer a patient's queries satisfactorily. Information seemed to be valued for the respect it indicated that clinicians had for patients and how it was provided was an opportunity for practitioners to show empathy for a patient's concerns. This suggests that, for patients, cognitive approaches to trust which assume that trust is based on the deliberative consideration of evidence are less significant than affective approaches which are essentially non-rational. As Barbalet (2002) has argued, rational procedures such as performance data can help us to evaluate risks but they do not apply to circumstances in which trust is most important since these typically concern areas of uncertainty where the capacity of reason to resolve the issue is limited. Yet, as Brown (2008: 21), drawing on the work of Habermas, suggests:

> The inherently instrumental rationality of auditing/account-ability mechanisms is unable to comprehend or measure the human aspects of health care. Rather the personal, tacit experience of doctors and the concerns of the person become the pollutants, the sewerage of emotionality, which are filtered off and where audit economic and risk focused instrumentality becomes the sole admissable value.

Our research did not investigate the impact of trust on health outcomes but it was evident that it has an indirect effect by encouraging patients to disclose sensitive information, which is needed for accurate diagnosis, and that it promotes concordance with medical advice. If patients do not trust a particular practitioner, they tend to take steps to avoid that particular individual, by for example waiting to see another clinician. Avoidance has not tended to be identified as a pattern of behaviour in theoretical models of patient participation. In arguably one of the most quoted classifications of participation, Hirshman (1970) distinguishes between exit, voice and loyalty, the first two options providing a means by which the public can influence producers. In this respect, patients in our study operated neither as 'economic man' in a consumer-characterized business-driven model of patient participation nor as 'political man' in a user-characterized democratically driven model of participation. Patients appear reluctant to exercise the exit option as practised by 'economic man' whose ability to change from one service to another will cause organizations to improve services. In fact, using private medicine was not associated with low trust; rather, it was undertaken mainly in order to reduce the waiting time for services. The voice option represents the political approach whereby users voice their dissatisfaction in order to gain improvements. The increasing number of complaints made against the NHS suggests that patients are increasingly willing to use this option. However, in our study rather than complain, patients tended to simply avoid the person they distrusted, seeking out another practitioner. Loyalty affects individual decisions by making voice rather than exit more probable, all things being equal. Barry (1974) has criticized Hirshman's model for ignoring a third and potentially more relevant option: silent non-exit. Rather than expressing loyalty, silent non-exit may reflect the relative powerlessness of the public in the face of a complex modern bureaucracy and entrenched vested interests. However, our findings suggest that if silent non-exit takes the form of avoidance then patients do have a degree of power to obtain the type of care they want. Patients' preference for avoidance rather than voice suggests that the incidence of complaints and claims is not a useful indicator of trust in doctors as has been proposed (Allsop 2006). If it is used as such, it will significantly underestimate the extent to which people feel that trust has been misplaced and have taken steps to avoid the clinician or organization concerned.

Trust between patients and clinicians continues to be important in the therapeutic relationship but as this relationship has changed, trust is increasingly conditional and has to be earned by a clinician's care and competence.

INTER-PRACTITIONER TRUST

With the increasingly shared care approach to patient management, both within primary and secondary care, trust between clinicians is ever more salient, and reliability as well as honesty and competence are important components of trust. Our study supports Jackson et al.'s (2004) qualitative study of family doctors in Nova Scotia which reported that trust between providers developed over time through positive experiences. Clinicians' emphasis on the importance of honesty and openness to build trust was reported similarly in Hallas et al.'s (2004) survey which found that open and honest communication was associated with greater trust and mutual respect between paediatric nurse practitioners and US paediatricians. Trust was conditional in that it had to be earned although it was generally assumed that clinical colleagues would consider each other's interests and act with them in mind, except at the consultant level. As with patients, performance data appeared to have no influence on the extent of trust between clinicians; rather trust was earned through clinical interactions and communication which acted as opportunities to demonstrate competence, honesty and reliability.

Table 6.1 summarizes the types of behaviour that clinicians demonstrate when they trust or distrust other practitioners. Like patients, they will also avoid a clinician who they do not trust, either trying to avoid referrals to them or seeking alternative clinical opinions to check their advice. Trust is also shown in the degree of delegation and supervision that senior clinicians feel is necessary and possible.

Table 6.1 High and low trust behaviour as identified by clinicians

High trust behaviour	Low trust behaviour
Limited supervision and checking that work has been done	Constant monitoring and increased supervision
Delegation of patient management	Limit clinical involvement
Significant professional autonomy	Little delegation of authority
Not anxious about holiday cover	Concerned by cover
Praise patient management	Criticize patient management
Seek advice from a particular clinician	Avoid asking advice from a particular clinician
Accept clinical opinion	Seek another clinical opinion
Openly seek help with a task that is beyond your clinical competence	Do not voice concerns about your competence to do a given task or seek support
Raise concerns directly and informally with a colleague or discuss first with peers	Speak to senior clinician about concerns regarding a colleague or use formal complaints procedure
Good communication, informal and unwritten	Poor communication, often formal and written
Good teamworking	Poor teamworking

Mutual trust between practitioners is demonstrated by the extent to which they will support each other and whether they are happy to leave a patient in the other's care. As Fox (1974) proposed in his book about work roles and trust relations, trust between practitioners is demonstrated when limited constraints are put on each other's discretion to act. In the surgical teams junior doctors were given a narrow task range and carefully defined role at the beginning of their training period but as more senior clinicians came to trust their competence and reliability, their task range widened and their role was more diffusely defined. In this respect trust appears to be important for more efficient working within healthcare as delegation of tasks and teamworking are essential in the modern delivery of health services. The consequences of better teamworking also impact on patient care and serve to link inter-practitioner trust with patient trust as depicted in Figure 6.2.

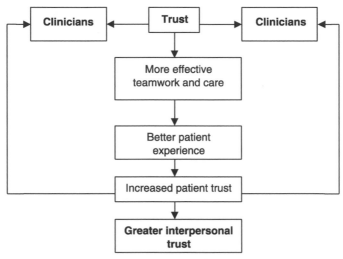

Figure 6.2 Reframing trust relationships: the links between inter-practitioner and patient trust

TRUST IN HEALTHCARE MANAGERS

Clinicians' and patients' trust in managers is similarly conditional in that it has to be earned. The relationship between clinicians and managers is increasingly interdependent with managers relying on clinicians to deliver services efficiently and effectively so that they can meet central targets, such as those relating to waiting times and clinicians relying on managers to obtain the resources they need to provide and enhance services. In this context trust is very important but we found distinct differences in the nature of trust relations according to the organizational setting. In primary care where management involvement in the delivery of clinical services is more limited, a certain degree of mutual trust had been achieved between primary care trust (PCT) managers and clinicians, albeit with continued reservations from GPs as to the PCT agenda and the extent to which it reflects their interests. There was a sense of local managers and clinicians working together to try to meet government requirements and align them with practices' clinical priorities and interests. In contrast, in the secondary care case study where managers sought greater influence over clinical activity, we found that distrust rather than trust was pervasive. Clinicians will not trust managers if they perceive them as being motivated by different interests and having values that conflict with the needs of clinical care. If managers fail to deliver what was promised, either because they were not honest about their ability to secure the necessary resources or were simply incompetent, then trust will be lost.

Our findings do suggest that trust in managers can be earned. In addition to showing some degree of common interest, managers need to be accessible and visible, as well as honest and competent. The approach of clinical managers appears to be more constructive in promoting trust; their presence on the wards and rapport with clinical staff encouraging clinicians to seek their support in tackling problems. Where there is trust between managers and practitioners, this offers organizational benefits in terms of better working relations, improved retention of staff and faster resolution of problems. The director of nursing talked about how nurses were willing to confide in her and seek her support in overcoming problems because she was trusted. As in patient and clinical relationships, where managers are not trusted clinicians will try to avoid them, and where communication is necessary this is likely to be more formal and in writing. In contrast, high trust between managers and clinicians is reflected in lower levels of monitoring, checking of activity and more honest and open communication. Patients tend not to have a relationship with managers but many decide whether they trust them based on the cleanliness of the hospitals and clinics they attend. Hygiene is an indicator of managerial competence and where this is considered poor, patients reason that they cannot trust managers to be effective in other areas of health service delivery.

THE EXPLANATORY POWER OF THE THEORETICAL FRAMEWORK

What then are the implications of these findings for theory, and does our framework and the types of relationship depicted in it have any explanatory power? Our research appears to confirm that the nature of trust relationships is affected by the broader organizational context in which health services are delivered. Macro-level changes, in terms of greater expectations of patient self-management and increased patient participation in decision-making, together with broader social changes with regard to reduced deference towards experts have created changes in trust between patients and clinicians. The increasing partnership between patients and clinicians in managing health problems and the greater interdependence of clinicians and managers in providing multidisciplinary shared care have changed how patients, clinicians and managers trust each other. However, at the micro level there were more similarities than differences in the nature of trust according to organizational setting. Although we expected patients with a long-term condition treated in primary care to require more mutual trust, and that patients with a more complex condition in an acute setting would show less conditional trust, in fact both groups of patients wanted mutual trust and trust was largely earned. It may be that the extent that trust is conditional is more a product of the nature of the patient's illness rather than the organizational setting. Mechanic and Meyer's (2000) research in the US found that patients with breast cancer appeared to have the highest level of trust, in part because of the life-threatening nature of the illness, compared with those with other conditions. Although the hip replacement patients in our research were undergoing acute care, making them more dependent on clinical competence, the elective nature of their treatment and the importance of their contribution to rehabilitation meant that trust was largely conditional once they were through surgery. Research with unelective trauma patients, admitted through Accident & Emergency, might have shown much greater forced trust or blind trust rather than conditional trust. What is consistent with our study and Mechanic's research is that the patient experience is fundamental to trust generation. In his study patients with Lyme disease talked about their loss of trust due to the difficulties they had experienced in obtaining a diagnosis.

As a result of these findings we have revised our theoretical framework (see Table 6.2). Our original proposition that information would be important in trust creation has been shown to have limited explanatory power. As Kuhlmann (2006) has suggested, there does appear to be a shift away from trust in individual qualifications and embodied practices but we would argue not from trust in information obtained from scientific-bureaucratic . measurements or assessments. Trust is conditional and has to be earned but the sources of trust are the quality of the patient–clinician interaction, the competence and empathy that is displayed, rather than abstract disembodied data. Thus, it is earned trust conditional on experience rather than informed trust which was meaningful in these different contexts. Patients do not demand 'proof' of trustworthiness; rather they assess for themselves the quality of service provision based on their personal experience of care. This notion of earned trust

Table 6.2 Revised theoretical framework

Relationship	Trustor		Trustee		Context	Type of trust
	Affect-based	Cognition-based	Assumed trust based on status	Earned trust		
Traditional clinician–patient	X		X		Paternalistic medicine	Embodied trust
New NHS clinician–patient	X	X	In a minority of patients	Earned through competence and experience of care	Mutual trust and patient partnership in primary care / Forced mutual trust in secondary care	Embodied trust / Conditional trust
Traditional clinician–clinician		X	X		Autonomous individualized care	Peer trust
New NHS clinician–clinician		X	In a minority of junior doctors	Earned through honesty, reliability and competence	Shared care	Conditional trust
Traditional clinician–manager	X		X		Administrative support for autonomous professionals	Status trust
New NHS clinician–manager		X		Earned through altruism, accessibility, visibility, honesty and competence	Active management including use of performance targets	Conditional trust

appears to be similar to the idea of active trust which is believed to be a new form of trust emerging within modernity (Giddens 1994). Active trust emerged from the so-called 'cultural turn' away from received authority and expertise towards a critical citizenry. It has to be won and cannot be taken for granted as it is not now based on status and deference to accredited experts (Zinn and Taylor-Gooby 2006).

Likewise, in inter-practitioner relationships and clinician-manager relations, trust is the product of human interaction, with each encounter adding to or diminishing levels of trust between individuals. Figure 6.3 illustrates the conditionality of interpersonal trust in healthcare relationships. Trust can no longer be assumed, based on professional status and seniority; instead it is conditional and is earned through a variety of strategies that demonstrate honesty, reliability, competence, accessibility and that colleagues share similar values and will look after each other's interests. Thus, the performance of the manager is assessed and earned in terms of these strategies rather than judgements about performance based on more 'objective' and abstract data.

The findings of our study can be contrasted with Robb and Greenhalgh's (2006) analysis of narratives of interpreted consultations in primary care which is informed by critical theory. They begin to tease out the relationship between institutional and interpersonal

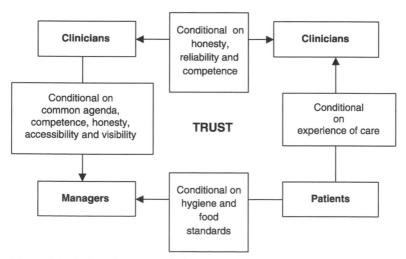

Figure 6.3 Reframing trust relationships in healthcare: the conditionality of interpersonal trust

trust through the use of three concepts of trust: voluntary, coercive and hegemonic, which they argue apply to both the macro and micro levels. Central to their theoretical approach are different dimensions of power which they argue can be both identifiable and invisible. They draw on Weberian concepts of bureaucracy and Habermasian concepts of communicative and strategic action to develop their typology, and suggest voluntary trust at both interpersonal and institutional levels is or would be associated with a more open communicative strategy in the interaction in the consultation. The three types of trust were found to exist in different components of the triadic relationships but coercive and hegemonic trust dominated, which had an impact on the nature of communication which tended to be strategic and on the outcome of the consultation. In contrast, patients in our study appeared to hold a degree of power, particularly those in primary care where their relationship with clinicians in the practice was more negotiated, hence their trust was voluntary but conditional. Their analysis raises the question about how 'informed' or 'conditional' trust might manifest itself in the clinician–patient relationship given the prevalence of coercive and hegemonic trust rather than voluntary trust. This question needs to be further explored in other clinical and organizational settings with patients from different backgrounds.

There is also the question of the extent to which and how trust relations have changed? The conceptual framework developed here was derived primarily from theory as there is a lack of empirical evidence particularly about trust relations at the organizational and institutional levels and about if and how these trust relations may have changed. Our study in the two different clinical and organizational settings had a cross-sectional design and any accounts of change were derived from retrospective narratives rather than evidence from a prospective longitudinal study interviewing different cohorts of informants at different points in time. It could be argued that conditional trust grounded in experience rather than assumed or blind trust has always been the most common form of trust relations. In the same way as the assumed passivity and acquiescence of the patient in studies of provider–patient relationships may have reflected the influence of a managerial perspective and a methodological approach dominated by surveys (Williams and Calnan 1996), then the depiction of patient passivity in trust relations may be primarily a product of sociological, professional and policy discourses. The qualitative data derived from our research does at least provide an indication of the nature of trust relationships in the NHS in the first decade of the twenty-first century and as such could be used in subsequent studies when examining how trust is changing.

It is clearly evident from our study that trust matters in healthcare relationships in the NHS. Trust also continues to be salient to the UK policy agenda. Lord Darzi, in his 2007 review of the NHS, identified trust as being an important attribute of the UK's system of primary healthcare:

> In my visits around the country, I have witnessed for myself the strength of our primary care and community services. Our registered GP list system is renowned internationally. Our primary care system co-ordinates care for patients in a way few other countries match. There are strong bonds of trust between staff and their patients, families and carers.
>
> (Darzi 2007: 24)

Despite this, our research suggests that the creation and maintenance of trust may be at odds with government health policies such as the promotion of patient choice (Department of Health 2004b) and the use of targets and performance management to achieve accountability. In the next section we examine how what we know about trust and how it is built and lost conflicts with certain aspects of current health policy.

IMPLICATIONS FOR POLICY: ACCOUNTABILITY, PERFORMANCE MANAGEMENT AND TRUST

Concerns that public trust in healthcare institutions and in providers is under threat have led to policies aimed at improving the accountability of health professionals and local organizations through increased monitoring and reporting of performance. Such increased regulation has been promoted at the expense of trust which has been seen as obsolescent and risky (O'Neill 2004). However, the findings of our empirical research have not only highlighted the continued salience of trust to healthcare relationships but have questioned the effectiveness of performance management as a means of accountability and its ability to act as a marker of quality. Our research into trust suggests that performance data are not effective in providing assurance to service users regarding the quality of care provided by local health services. Harrison and Smith (2004) have argued that the new policy framework of clinical governance has sought to achieve a shift in focus from trust relationships between people to confidence in abstract systems, such as rules and regulations. The more behaviour is constrained by such systems so uncertainty is reduced and visibility is increased (Giddens 1990), the less we need to rely on trust (Smith 2001). However, our research suggests that patients and practitioners do not find current external performance measurements credible. In both case studies healthcare professionals reported that such data did not accurately reflect the quality of care provided by individual practitioners and clinical teams. Patients considered performance data to be unreliable as they were open to manipulation by managers. This supports the findings of other studies that have evaluated the impact of external performance measures. Mannion and Goddard's (2003) evaluation of the impact of the CRAG clinical outcome indicators in Scotland reported limited use of such data by patients and GPs and also within hospital trusts. Similarly, studies of the use of US report cards have found on the whole that published performance rarely stimulates quality improvement (Marshall et al. 2000) and the public distrusts and fails to make use of it (Schneider and Lieberman 2001).

We found that trust is influenced by performance in terms of patients' experience of care but not necessarily by performance indicators. This gives weight to Power's (1997) argument that the growth of performance measurement and audit may merely result in 'certificates of comfort' offering reassurance that performance is being measured without resulting in change. Where trust is low the reliability of information published may be questioned and any uncertainty in the data and what it means may further undermine public confidence. If performance measures such as star ratings are ineffective in building up confidence in organizations, then institutional as well as interpersonal trust remains important.

Our research also highlighted that the use of performance management can be detrimental to relationships between clinicians and managers and damaging to trust. One of the key reasons for distrust in clinician–manager relationships was the imposition of top-down targets in terms of service delivery, which seemed to be at odds with clinicians' agenda to provide high quality care based on clinical need. Furthermore, both managers and clinicians considered that performance management involved such a burden of monitoring and reporting of activity and chasing to attain targets that there was little capacity for strategic development of services. Patients also criticized targets for their negative impact on care:

What about trust in the NHS? I mean do you trust the NHS?
Diabetes patient: Well I did have great trust in them, but now it
seems that they are on to a bottom line, everybody has to meet a
– what is it they call it, they have to meet a?
These targets?
Yeah targets, that's right, everything is targeted now, which
I think is wrong. It's taking everything away from doctors,
they have to rush things through, if they have to see ten patients
an hour then they have to see then patients an hour, where
sometimes it's not practical.

The low trust associated with performance management that we
found in our case studies appears to have been reported more
widely. In Lord Darzi's (2007: 5) review of the NHS he reported
that:

> Some staff tell me that they haven't been listened to and trusted.
> They do not feel that their values – including wanting to
> improve the quality of care have been fully recognized. Nor do
> they feel that they have always been given the credit for the
> improvements that have been made.

In contrast, trust appears to offer significant organizational benefits.
Our research supports the findings of other studies that have considered the impact of trust on workplace relations in healthcare
settings, in that trust encouraged collaborative practice between clinicians, was associated with job satisfaction and motivation, and
reduced transaction costs due to lower surveillance and monitoring
costs and the general enhancement of efficiency. Performance management has been successful in focusing managerial and clinical
attention on reducing waiting times but from a patient perspective in
its current form, it is not a meaningful tool for ensuring the accountability of healthcare organizations or an effective substitution for
trust. It may be an effective mechanism for obtaining internal
accountability up to the centre but it appears to be harmful to hori-
zontal accountability between clinical and managerial peers and
outwards in terms of accountability to patients and the public.
The perverse effects of performance management mean that policy
makers and health service managers need to look again at how they
can achieve meaningful accountability which supports public trust in
healthcare organizations and the wider health system.

IMPLICATIONS FOR POLICY: TRUST
AND PATIENT CHOICE

Prior to our fieldwork we had proposed that patients' and their GPs' confidence in an organization might be influenced by performance data and that this might in turn affect choice of acute hospital for specialist services. Patients reported, at least in this study, that they were rarely actively involved in decisions about where to be referred to and performance data were only drawn upon to check out the doctor or organization after a referral decision was made:

> Hip patient 11: What choice does a layman have? To have choice, to exercise choice, you need knowledge and we do not have that so when I was told who the surgeon would be, whose team I was going to be referred to I then started searching on the Internet. There is a web site that gives you the star ratings of the various hospitals. Dr A came up very well and after talking to friends it appears that by chance I have landed at the door of the top hip man so I was very happy about that and fortunate.

The reputation of and relationship with the surgeon, derived mainly from experiential knowledge, seemed to be important even where choice was perceived to be available.

> Patient 3: They did write to me to ask if I would be prepared to change my surgeon and to go to hospital C and I did say I would go to hospital C but I would not change my surgeon . . . I have been with Dr A from the start and that was where my confidence lay.

> Patient 4: No choice but if I had I would have gone to hospital B because I have heard so much. It would have been a so and so to have to wait and if they had said hospital C or anything like that I would have tried to hang on to Dr B . . . well if you have a surgeon with a big reputation then that would be the first thing.

However, this reputation seems to embrace trust in the team as a whole:

> Patient 7: Oh the consultant, I do not know if I actually met him but I met part of his team. I expect to see one of his reps and for him to tell me the facts. I do not necessarily need to see the man himself, and well, waste the man's time.

Hospitals were assessed both in terms of the type of service they provide and levels of hygiene although these assessments appeared to be based once again mainly on experiential knowledge.

> Hip patient 7: Well I have not been impressed with what goes on at hospital A myself. Well my brother was in there and I felt it was a very dirty hospital, not very clean.

> Patient 11: I had a choice of hospital B or C and chose B. Well for a start they have a lot of surgeons coming in from abroad so the after care is not provided . . . and I do not feel fast track surgery is a good idea . . . and I had already been going to hospital B so I felt it was easier to go there.

In contrast, practitioners did think that performance information as reported in the media might have an influence on patients' assessment:

> Research fellow: The trust ratings come out and you will get the local papers which say 'we have got the worst hospitals in the country' which was awful for the patients up until recently, where they have not had a choice as these are their hospitals and they are stuck with them. I think then you get the feeling that when you see patients in the clinic they say 'God, they're right this place is dirty' whereas if you get a better rating the next year they come in and say 'I will tell you what it's really nice and clean' and you know full well the cleaning standards have not changed in the last year.

Choice and trust do seem to be related and when choice is exercised, it does seem to be based on trust of the doctors' competence and the cleanliness of the hospital, mainly derived from indirect or direct experience. Performance information appears to act post the referral decision to influence the extent to which patients feel comfortable with the referral rather than actively determining where patients choose to be referred (see Figure 6.4).

TRUST AND QUALITY OF CARE

Our research suggests that institutional trust and patients' trust in clinicians is a product of the patient experience of care; when patients have a positive experience of care trust is high and when they experience problems with health services trust is lower. Other research has reported that high-quality doctor–patient interactions

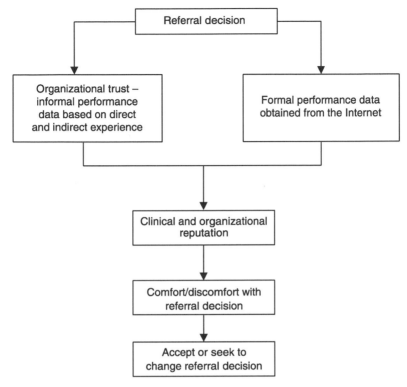

Figure 6.4   Trust and choice at the point of referral

are characterized by high levels of trust and that high levels of trust are associated with high-quality care (Caterinicchhio 1979; Walker and Brooksby 1998; Joffe et al. 2003). Thom et al.'s (2004) research in the US has caused them to suggest that levels of trust might be a more sensitive indicator of performance than patient satisfaction. Such a comparison was not made in this study, although given the increasing emphasis in patients' accounts of earned trust, it appears that assessments of trust might be more closely tied with performance than they were in the past, and also more closely linked with assessments of satisfaction which are believed to be based on recent past performance. For example:

Hip patient 1: You hear a lot of things and I must speak honestly, my experience whilst I was in hospital B was no problems at all. When I had the first hip operation a young doctor came in, and anything I wanted to know he was willing to tell me, even to the point that they did warn me before the operation that I could have a slight problem with feeling in my leg . . . I had no complaints about the nurses or the way I was treated in hospital at all.

Hip patient 3: I think as far as hospital B is concerned I do not think there is too much they could do as the treatment that I received and the food was good . . . it wasn't obviously up to hotel or home standard but it was good. For example, on one Sunday morning the cleaning supervisor came in and told one of the girls to get round and do under the beds again. . I think the staff did their job, they were careful and very competent and food and cleanliness were good. I have no complaints but with no experience of any hospital I cannot really judge.

These patients present mainly positive accounts of their experience of hospital for hip surgery which influences both assessments of satisfaction and the maintenance or enhancement of trust.

INSTITUTIONAL TRUST

In recent years policy makers have expressed widespread concern about declining institutional trust. The Cabinet Office Strategy Unit report on Risk notes that a wide range of UK institutions have suffered a significant drop in trust over the past two decades (COSU 2002) and it appears to be a trend which is not restricted to the UK (OECD 2001). This was also evident in results from the 2001 BSA survey which showed that over 40 per cent of respondents thought that they would not trust NHS hospitals to spend their money wisely in the interest of patients (Taylor-Gooby 2008). The findings of our research appear to support this view. While patients expressed high levels of trust in their GP and the GP practice or the surgical team in hospital, they tended to be less positive about the NHS in general. Hall's (2006) survey of HMO members found that system trust could help the development of interpersonal trust, without prior knowledge of the individual clinician, but it is not known how clinician–patient trust affects institutional trust. In our study patients' trust in their GPs encouraged them to speak favourably about the practice but it did not translate into increased trust of the health service as a whole. In fact, one patient did not regard their

GP as part of the wider NHS, perceiving him more as an important figure within the community:

> *So if you take the NHS as a whole, would you say that your level of trust in it generally has changed at all?*
> Diabetes patient: Well my own personal experience, of course, I haven't had any.
> *Right yes, other than obviously with your GP.*
> Yeah, and funnily enough I don't think of that as the NHS.
> *Right, now why is that?*
> Never have done, because it's something we've always had, isn't it, before the National Health? Well not before the National Health Service – yeah I can remember going to a doctor and having to pay 5 shillings to see him. I can remember that. Um but a GP is part of the community.
> *Right.*
> Like the vicar isn't he?

Two of the clinicians were not certain that public trust in the NHS had fallen and that there would always be those who praise the NHS and those who criticize it, possibly reflecting whether they have had emergency or pre-elective care.

> Diabetes nurse: It's interesting, because patients come in who have had to go into secondary care for whatever reason, and if they've been really, really poorly and it's been an emergency, they come out and they say, 'People may knock the NHS, but thank God for the NHS.' Um but patients that go in for pre-booked operations like hips and things come out moaning like anything. And I think the general consensus is, 'The NHS is there when you need it, thank God for it, we're lucky to have it. But actually, you know, it is pretty dirty and [laughs] disgusting.'

In this way, the patient's experience of care acts to link interpersonal trust with organizational and institutional trust (see Figure 6.5).

In our study those hip patients who had experienced good care within the hospital spoke in positive terms about the surgical team and would be happy to be referred there again for surgery, but this did not mean that they trusted the hospital more widely to provide good care. Trust is a product of human interaction and as a result institutional trust appears to be limited to that section of the service that has provided patients with good care. This appears to resonate with the pattern of findings from a recent analysis of the British Social Attitudes data (Taylor-Gooby 2008) which show that

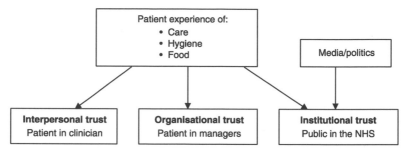

Figure 6.5   Reframing trust relationships in healthcare: the links between patient experience and interpersonal, organizational and institutional trust

rational/objective and affectual/subjective factors contribute to public trust in the NHS. The extent to which the service treats its users in ways that indicate it respects their interests is important, alongside perceptions of more objective factors such as staffing levels and quality of treatment. This, according to Taylor-Gooby (2008), reflects a general conclusion from empirical research that trust is derived from two analytically separate bases: cognitive deliberative, rational considerations of track-record based on good information and a more affective acceptance that the trustee shares values and interests with the trustor.

Trust in the NHS was also linked to patients' views of NHS managers and their competence to organize services. Reforms to the delivery of services may have improved performance in terms of reduced waiting times but patients will not be satisfied if when they go into hospital they find it dirty or the staff too rushed to help. Managers reported that the low level of public trust in NHS managers related to media portrayals of them as faceless bureaucrats, responsible for diverting resources from patient care. However, while patients may be influenced by media criticism that there are too many managers, their distrust of them appears to relate to their personal experience of services and managers' competence in ensuring that hospitals are clean and have appropriate standards of hygiene.

Do you think the information provided in terms of star ratings can build patient trust in the NHS and the quality of care they can expect?
Practice manager: Er, I think it can. But at the end of the day the anecdote is still very powerful, and whether it's your neighbour or your relative. And, you know, a single good experience, I

think, in somebody's mind will kind of override any statistics you give them . . . And I think this will always be the case. And you know, we've all got experience of the NHS. And I think that's what, in my view, that's what's the most powerful thing for people.

Given that the patient experience appears to be the most important contributor to patient trust or distrust in a particular healthcare organization, if hospitals wish to increase trust in them then they will need to ensure that all aspects of the patient's stay are positive, from the cleanliness of the wards and public spaces to whether they are treated with dignity and respect by clinical staff. Seeking patient views and involving them in decisions about services is important if organizations are going to capture patient priorities. Likewise, exploring complaints and identifying system level failings is necessary to ensure that negative aspects of a patient's care are acted upon. As the personal anecdote appears to be so strong in shaping public opinion, organizations need to identify whether their staff are acting as advocates or critics of the institution as their views will carry particular weight with patients. Open and honest communication will encourage patients and healthcare practitioners to trust in a particular organization if managers also visibly demonstrate their competence by maintaining high standards of hygiene and by delivering on what was promised. The steps that hospital managers could take to increase organizational trust might in turn create increased institutional trust in the NHS. Figure 6.6 shows how the source of institutional trust links through organizational trust back to the individual patient experience.

AN AGENDA FOR FUTURE RESEARCH

Despite the exploratory nature of our empirical research, its clear finding that trust continues to be relevant and important to healthcare relationships suggests that further research into trust in healthcare is merited. In this final section we propose an agenda for future research.

Trust in different healthcare relationships

Most of the research relating to trust in healthcare contexts has focused on patients' trust in health professionals. However, the trust

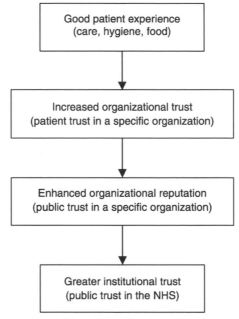

Figure 6.6   Generation of institutional trust

that patients (and, more broadly, members of the public) express and place in healthcare teams, healthcare provider organizations, healthcare practitioners and possibly broader systems of healthcare financing, provision and regulation, warrant further attention than they have been paid to date. Our research suggests that the individual patient experience and the trust that people place in individual healthcare professionals is linked to institutional trust in healthcare organizations, professions or systems but how one interacts with the other warrants further research. Such studies might facilitate understanding of the various claims and counter claims that are made about the so-called erosion of public trust in medicine and other healthcare institutions (Calnan et al. 2006a).

Questions also need to be asked about whether, and if so how, trust in healthcare organizations and systems is related to the ways in which healthcare is financed and organized. Does this, and how does this, vary according to individuals' status, political opinions and loyalties? For example, are people who have direct use of health services more trusting, and does this depend on their satisfaction with their healthcare experiences?

Trust relationships between healthcare providers, for example in the NHS between general practitioners and hospital doctors, and between clinicians and managers, also appear to have been under-researched. It is not clear why they have been neglected, although one possible explanation is that the relationships are not seen to be problematic or important in terms of consequences for care. Such an assertion is contradicted by Gilson (2006) who suggests that managers' treatment of providers can affect providers' treatment of patients, and that managerial behaviour and practices set the rules and norms that shape provider behaviour. Gilson argues that manager–provider relationships will be particularly important for low- and middle-income countries, where issues of human resource management in health services has virtually been ignored to date.

In the UK, our research into clinician–managerial relationships and the developing roles of clinical managers make research into trust between managers and providers and its potential impact on quality of care highly pertinent. How does inter-managerial trust operate between senior and middle healthcare managers and how does that impact on clinician–manager relations? The strains and tensions between GPs and hospital doctors, and doctors and managers, have been well documented, but questions about the implications of trust, or the lack of it, in these relationships have yet to be fully answered.

The implications of trust

The second theme for future research (Calnan et al. 2006a) focuses on the implications of trust for important healthcare processes and outcomes. Although trust may have an intrinsic value, interest is more often focused on its possible instrumental value. The implications of trust may be extremely far reaching. For example, as Gilson (2006) suggests, trust relations between citizens and health systems may, in some contexts, provide an opportunity to build civic trust with a much wider social value. More usually, considerations of the implications of trust focus on questions about whether and how trust relations impinge on healthcare outcomes. These questions can be asked about trust relations between patients and their healthcare providers (at both micro and macro levels) and about trust relations between healthcare professionals within healthcare organizations.

It is still not clear whether particular forms and levels of trust between patients and their healthcare providers have benefits for patients in terms of improved clinical and health status outcomes and, if so, how these effects might be mediated. Entwistle and Quick (2006) highlight the uncertainty about whether and how patients' trust in their healthcare providers might in practice make them more or less likely to be vigilant about the possibility of errors in their healthcare, and thus more or less susceptible to iatrogenic harm. Also, as has been suggested, the trust that patients place in healthcare providers may be more or less active and informed, with potentially different consequences for the kinds of choice and contribution that patients are able and willing to make in relation to their healthcare, and thus to their healthcare outcomes. These and other possible pathways between trust and health, including the possibility that trust has direct therapeutic benefits and is key to the placebo effect, need to be examined. Some of the potential dangers of blind trust have been identified and in some contexts lower levels of trust may be both understandable and appropriate. However, the key questions are what levels and types of trust contribute to positive health outcomes and effective healthcare delivery and whether positive outcomes for the organization are compatible with positive outcomes for the patient and the clinician. This is linked to the question raised about what kind of trust relations are compatible with empowerment or whether these two concepts are at odds with one another.

In terms of trust relations among and between healthcare professionals and managers within healthcare provider organizations, there are important questions to be investigated about the relationships between trust and performance, and particularly trust and the implementation of changes to organizational structures and approaches to healthcare delivery. Organizational research in other settings has shown that trust is important for group cohesion, teamworking, job satisfaction and organizational efficiency, but questions about the ways in which trust might contribute to the effectiveness of health service provision, and how it might be built and sustained, have been relatively neglected even though they are highly salient for health service managers.

The role of trust in the context of efforts to implement changes in service delivery and/or the introduction of innovative technologies also warrants assessment. Questions arise, for example, about the formation and implications of trust in local 'product champions' and other 'brokers of change and knowledge', and in other sources of information and advice, including the kinds of summaries of research findings and clinical practice guidelines that are disseminated as part of the drive towards evidence-based practice. There are also still questions to be asked about whether and how things other than persons might be trusted, and how trust in these is mediated by interpersonal contact.

Complaints from patients have sometimes been used as an indicator of the performance of healthcare organizations and this raises questions about the relationship between trust, medical errors and complaints. Our research suggests that there is not necessarily a linear and simple inverse relationship between trust and complaints: a high level of complaints reflects a low level of trust. Low levels of trust among our respondents resulted in avoidance instead of complaints. There is a need to examine in what contexts mistakes lead to a loss of trust resulting in avoidance, in what contexts mistakes result in complaints or even intense blame, and when errors are forgiven and do not diminish trust. There is also the broader question about how the nature of complaints and their presentation affect public levels of trust in the medical profession as an institution and the wider health system (Allsop 2006).

Contexts and circumstances

The third theme (Calnan et al. 2006a) examines the importance of contexts and circumstances in influencing the salience, domains, levels and appropriateness of trust. Our exploratory study suggests that innovations in service delivery in the UK, such as walk-in clinics and specialist open-access clinics in primary care have changed, but not undermined, patient–clinician trust relations, traditionally claimed to be based on continuity of care and associated with general practitioners. A key question that needs to be further explored is whether and how trust relations vary according to different clinical conditions. In conditions where there is considerable uncertainty about outcomes such as the treatment of cancer, 'mutual trust' which was reported by patients in our study may be less relevant to patients who may take or have to take a more 'passive' role, and higher levels of trust or different trust relations may emerge. Trust may be particularly pertinent for patients with mental health problems with concerns about confidentiality because of the stigma and because trusting relationships may be the actual modes of treatment (e.g. psychotherapy) and therefore may be critical to therapeutic outcomes. In the management of sometimes long-term complex conditions like cancer and mental health, do trust relations between patients and clinicians change, and if so how?

The context of chronic illness appears to raise a further set of issues which relate to trust. The enhanced knowledge, experience and expertise of some people with chronic illness may increase their awareness of both the benefits and the risks and limitations of modern scientific medicine and technology. Consequently, they may have an increased awareness of the possible risks and harm of certain orthodox medications and possibly inclined to be attracted to and trust in complementary treatments which are perceived as less harmful and safer because they are more 'natural'. This is particularly salient where discreet pathology is more elusive such as with some chronic illnesses.

The above discussion about the attractions of complementary medicine shows how it is sometimes difficult to disentangle beliefs about trust in scientific medicine from beliefs about trust in medical professionals. However, a more 'straightforward' example is the debate about MMR which has been amplified in the media (Hobson-West 2007). The focus here was on confidence in the 'scientific' evidence as well as trust in the purveyors of this evidence. Are government sources of evidence more trustworthy than professional sources? This also raises the general question of the relationship between confidence and trust. It is clearly possible to have low confidence in the system but high trust in the practitioner that specifically provides the service, but how do the two concepts relate to one another? For example, in this study assessments of competence both by practitioners and patients were embedded in and formed part of judgements about trust. Other technologies also have implications for issues of trust such as the developments in molecular genetics and the increased use of genetic testing and therapy and the use of DNA which may affect trust between the patient and clinician and between family members. These technologies' capacity to intervene at a fundamental level of human biology has given rise to increased awareness of risk and uncertainty about the consequences of such interventions and specific concerns about ethical issues and the social implications of the new genetics (Calnan et al. 2006b).

What of the diverse social and economic circumstances in which people live and their possible impact and consequences for trust relations? Does gender, socio-economic status or age of the patient influence the nature of interpersonal relations with clinicians?

There is also the broader question of how trust relations in healthcare compare with those in other sections of welfare and public sector services. Have the unique characteristics of the healthcare setting proved more resistant to organizational and social change, which may have eroded or changed trust relations in other settings, or is 'conditional trust' now common in service provision throughout the public sector? There is also the question of whether trust is still as politically salient now as it was in the late 1990s. The current direction of UK government policy with its emphasis on individual choice and the marketization of public services may have a cumulative negative impact on social capital through its influence on citizenship and participation and intra-agency and inter-agency cooperation. This returns us to the question of the nature of the relationship between interpersonal and institutional trust, and whether in the context of patient choice of provider healthcare, managers will perceive a value in fostering public trust in their organization and the clinicians they employ. In this context the potential financial implications of consumer choice may increase the salience of trust and may stimulate research to better understand the nature of institutional trust and how it links to the individual patient's experience of clinical care.

Conceptualising trust

Finally, research investigating trust will depend on the way it is conceptualized (Calnan et al. 2006a). Hence, the fourth thematic area involves the conceptualization of trust and how differences in the way it is conceptualized may have important implications for how to operationalize and measure it. Our findings suggest that how trust can be built (and lost) does depend on how individuals conceptualize it. Although certain dimensions of trust such as competence were important to all respondents in our study, there was also significant variation in managers', patients' and clinicians' understanding of trust and its determinants. It is important when developing instruments to measure trust to reflect this variation in any trust scales. In our study we also sought to distinguish between beliefs and behaviour or felt and enacted trust and to explore this relationship empirically. Informants reported many examples of the high and low trust behaviours we proposed in Chapter 2 (see page 53), and as such this information could be usefully applied when developing trust measures.

Methodologically, we found it harder to tap into beliefs or felt trust; informants only identified suspicion of others' motives and a belief that others might harm them as attitudes that reflected felt trust. Further empirical research is needed to explore whether there are other attitudes that more closely reflect felt trust and, if so, whether there is a direct relationship between trust beliefs and behaviour. In our study where there was active distrust between clinicians and managers, the former were suspicious of managers' intentions resulting in formal methods of communication and avoidance behaviour. It would be interesting to identify in other contexts where trust or distrust is felt less intensely whether it necessarily results in such behaviours. Finally, there are a number of methodological questions about the design and methods to be used when investigating trust in empirical studies, not least of which is whether trust should be explored in similar ways across different settings.

CONCLUSIONS

A recurring theme throughout this book has been the continuing salience of trust to healthcare relations. Relationships between patients and clinicians, between practitioners and between clinicians and managers appear to be changing but trust, albeit in possibly new forms, is still highly relevant to both the therapeutic relationship and the effective delivery of healthcare. Levels of trust in healthcare professionals, both as individuals and institutions, remain high despite more open reporting of cases of medical negligence. Where patients have enjoyed a positive experience of care, trust in individual organizations and the wider NHS remains high. What then are the implications for broader policy and sociological discourses that paint a much gloomier picture of the role of trust in a post-modern society? One explanation for this disconnect between academic and policy discourses and the findings of empirical research may stem from differences in how trust is conceptualized. Social and cultural change may have produced a decline in embodied or blind trust (if it ever existed) but now conditional trust is more overtly evident; trust is still important for more questioning and less deferential patients but such trust has to be earned. Our empirical study into trust in healthcare relations in the NHS offers a marker for the nature of trust relations between patients, clinicians and managers against which future studies involving patients with different conditions, of different ages, in different clinical contexts, and in different healthcare systems can be compared.

APPENDIX: CASE STUDY SELECTION AND METHODS

The two case studies were carried out in a provincial city in southern England.

CASE STUDY 1: DIABETES

The case study focusing on type 2 diabetes was carried out in a large multi-partner, training general practice which served a deprived population in the suburb of the city. The patients with type 2 diabetes were selected according to the criteria listed below.

Patients listed on the practice diabetes register were classified as follows:

- Into two groups by age: 55–65 and 66+
- Into four groups by gender: male and female
- Into 12 sub-groups according to stage of treatment:

  ○ Early (diagnosed in last six months)
  ○ Medium (diagnosed between one and two years ago)
  ○ Late (diagnosed at least six years ago)

Two patients were randomly selected from each sub-group and invited for interview. Of the 24 invited 10 patients agreed to be interviewed, none had been diagnosed in the last 6 months (see Figure A.1 for the age, gender and occupational characteristics of the informants).

The healthcare clinicians and managers were selected purposively to reflect the provision of diabetes care in general practice. Six clinicians, one administrative member of staff and two managers agreed

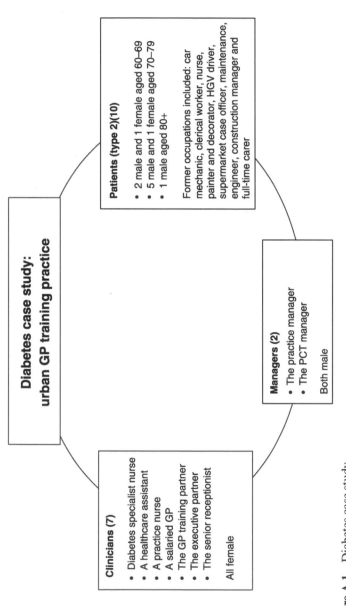

**Diabetes case study:
urban GP training practice**

Clinicians (7)
- Diabetes specialist nurse
- A healthcare assistant
- A practice nurse
- A salaried GP
- The GP training partner
- The executive partner
- The senior receptionist

All female

Managers (2)
- The practice manager
- The PCT manager

Both male

Patients (type 2)(10)
- 2 male and 1 female aged 60–69
- 5 male and 1 female aged 70–79
- 1 male aged 80+

Former occupations included: car
mechanic, clerical worker, nurse,
painter and decorator, HGV driver,
supermarket case officer, maintenance,
engineer, construction manager and
full-time carer

Figure A.1 Diabetes case study

to be interviewed (see Figure A.1 for distribution of types of clinician and manager interviewed).

CASE STUDY 2: HIP SURGERY

The second case study focused on elective hip surgery and was carried out in a specialist orthopaedic department in a city teaching hospital which served an urban population. Patients who had undergone hip surgery were selected from two surgical firms and 12 patients from each firm were invited to participate in the study. The patients were selected according to the following criteria:

All patients on the lists for elective hip or knee surgery with no co-morbidity who were having hip or knee surgery for the first time were identified from the clinic lists.

* This group was divided into three age groups:
  * Group A those aged under 55
  * Group B those aged between 55 and 65
  * Group C those aged over 65
* Each sub-group was then split into three categories according to their stage of treatment:
  * Early post-op (within three months of surgery)
  * Late post-op (at least three months post surgery)
This produced six different sub-groups of patients.
* Two patients, one male, one female were randomly selected from each of the six sub-groups

A letter was sent to each patient inviting them to take part in the study group, that is 24 in total with 12 from each of the two firms. Eleven agreed to be interviewed (six from one firm and five from the other). Figure A.2 shows the age, gender and occupational characteristics of the patients who took part in the study.

Healthcare practitioners and managers were selected purposively from the two surgical firms and the teams that worked with them. Fifteen clinicians, an administrative member of staff and two managers agreed to be interviewed. Figure A.2 shows the range and types of healthcare practitioner who were interviewed.

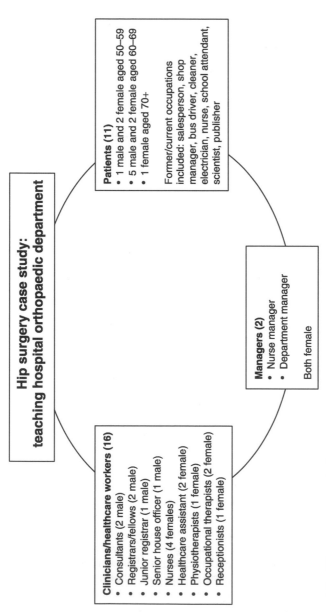

Hip surgery case study:
teaching hospital orthopaedic department

Clinicians/healthcare workers (16)
- Consultants (2 male)
- Registrars/fellows (2 male)
- Junior registrar (1 male)
- Senior house officer (1 male)
- Nurses (4 females)
- Healthcare assistant (2 female)
- Physiotherapists (1 female)
- Occupational therapists (2 female)
- Receptionists (1 female)

Managers (2)
- Nurse manager
- Department manager

Both female

Patients (11)
- 1 male and 2 female aged 50–59
- 5 male and 2 female aged 60–69
- 1 female aged 70+

Former/current occupations included: salesperson, shop manager, bus driver, cleaner, electrician, nurse, school attendant, scientist, publisher

Figure A.2   Hip surgery case study

Data collection

Qualitative methods are the most appropriate means of exploring informants' critical reasoning and experiences, particularly in exploratory research (Calnan and Ferlie, 2003). Thus, the primary method of data collection was informal face-to-face interviews which were carried out with key informants in the different settings. The bulk of the interviews were carried out by the authors although a PhD student trained in informal interviewing carried out some of the interviews with the patients. The interviews were carried out in 2006 and 2007.

Emphasis in the interviews was placed on spontaneous talk to allow subjects to describe their experiences, although the topic guides were linked to the conceptual framework which was developed to explain the development of new forms of trust relations in the NHS. This framework was described in Chapter 2 as were the typologies of the beliefs and behaviour which might characterize embodied as compared to informed trust for patients, peer as opposed to earned trust for clinicians, and status as compared with performance trust for managers. Thus, separate topic guides were developed for the patients, clinicians and managers, which consisted of a general discussion of their experiences as a patient in terms of their illness or condition, and the care and treatment they received or their experiences at work, and their roles and responsibilities followed by more specific focus on themes associated with trust. Each of the topic guides were piloted.

The interviews with patients with diabetes or who had hip surgery began with questions about their condition and the care they received, followed by exploring the thematic areas of information, decision-making behaviours that signal trust, what creates trust, the importance, benefits and problems of trust, others' intention and motivations and how individual trust might translate into institutional and organizational trust. A similar approach was taken for clinicians with interviews beginning with general questions about clinical practice, both past and present, and their management and treatment of diabetes or hip surgery, followed by the exploration of specific areas such as decision-making, the role of trust in successful clinical relations, clinical authority and reputation, performance assessment, information and behaviours that signal trust. Similar themes were explored with managers although the focus was on successful clinician–manager relations.

Data analysis

All face-to-face interviews were transcribed verbatim and the transcripts organized using Atlas/ti. A sequential analysis was conducted as the interviews progressed, allowing emergent themes to be addressed in later interviews. A provisional coding frame, derived from themes emerging from early stages of the research, was modified as the analysis proceeded and used to develop a theoretical framework that accounted for emerging themes. Samples of the transcripts were double-coded by the authors to assess reliability. To assist analysis, a thematic framework was developed, as described by Ritchie and Spencer (1994), using microsoft excel to chart data by theme, with cases kept in the same order for each subject chart to facilitate comparison between and within cases. Once charted the data were analysed, searching for patterns and associations and constantly comparing key themes.

Limitations of the study

The exploratory study was carried out in one general practice and one hospital department at one point in time. The general practice was a training practice and was part of a research network. The hospital department carried out research and medical training and was linked to a medical school. Quality of healthcare can be assessed in a number of different ways but judging from the patients' reports of both the general practice and the hospital department, the care provided was of a relatively high standard. This raises the question about how transferable the findings were to other organizational settings, particularly as the research was exploratory and in some respects innovative, and could not easily be compared to previously published work. It was shown that the salience and meaning of trust can be elicited from informants where trust levels are high. However, it might be important to examine trust in the context of lower quality of care as trust and quality are clearly closely related, and it might provide more concrete examples of where informants experienced a loss of trust. It might be argued that trust might be best explored when it is lost or under threat as like health, as opposed to illness, it is taken for granted, although this argument might not be as valid if according to our findings conditional or earned trust is now very prevalent. However, there is a clear need to carry out this research in other organizational settings to assess the extent to which the findings are transferable.

REFERENCES

Alaszweski, A. (2003) Risk, trust and health. *Health, Risk and Society*, 5(3): 235–40.

Allsop, J. (2006) Regaining trust in medicine: professional and state strategies, *Current Sociology*, 54(4): 621–36.

Altice, F., Mostashari, F. and Friedland, G. (2001) Trust and the acceptance of and adherence to antiretroviral therapy, *Journal of Acquired Immune Deficiency Syndromes*, 28(1): 47–58.

Anderson, L.A. and Dedrick, R.F. (1990) Development of the trust in physician scale: a measure to assess interpersonal trust in patient–physician relationships, *Psychological Reports*, 67: 1091–100.

Anheier, H.K. and Kendall, J. (2002) Interpersonal trust and voluntary associations, *British Journal of Sociology*, 53(3): 343–60.

Appleby, J. and Rosete, A. (2003) The NHS: keeping up with public expectations, in A. Park, J. Curtice, K. Thomson, L. Jarvis and C. Bromley (eds) *British Social Attitudes: The 20th Report – Continuity and Change Over Two Decades*, 20th edn. Sage: London.

Arksey, H. and Sloper, P. (1999) Disputed diagnoses: the cases of RSI and childhood cancer, *Social Science and Medicine*, 49: 483–97.

Baker, R., Mainous III, A.G., Pereira Gray, D. and Love, M.M. (2003) Exploration of the relationship between continuity, trust in regular doctors and patient satisfaction with consultations with family doctors, *Scandinavian Journal of Primary Health Care*, 21: 27–32.

Balkrishnan, R., Dugan, E., Carnacho, F.T. and Hall, M.A. (2003) Trust and satisfaction with physicians, insurers and the medical profession, *Medical Care*, 41(9): 1058–64.

Barbalet, J. (2002) *Emotions and Sociology*. Oxford: Blackwell Publishing.
Barbalet, J. (2005) Trust and uncertainty: the emotional basis of rationality. Paper presented at the ESRC RISK meeting, LSE, London, 15 December.
Barber, B. (1983) *The Logic and Limits of Trust*. New Brunswick, NJ: Rutgers University Press.
Barry, B. (1974) Review article: exit, voice and loyalty, *British Journal of Political Studies*, 4: 79–107.
Beck, U. (1992) *Risk Society*. London: Sage.
Booth, M., Bernard, D., Quine, S., Kang, M., Usherwood, T., Alperstein, G. and Bennett, D. (2004) Access to health care among Australian adolescents: young people's perspectives and their sociodemographic distribution, *Journal of Adolescent Health*, 34: 97–103.
Boulware, E.L., Ratner, L.E., Cooper, L.A., Sosa, J.A., La Veist, T.A. and Powe, N.R. (2002) Understanding disparities in donor behaviour: race and gender differences in willingness to donate blood and cadaveric organs, *Medical Care*, 40: 85–95.
Brereton, M. and Temple, M. (1999) The new public service ethos: an ethical environment for governance, *Public Administration*, 77(3): 455–74.
Brown, P. (2008) Trusting in the new NHS: instrumental or communicative action, *Sociology of Health and Illness*, 30: 349–363.
Burkitt Wright, E., Holcombe, C. and Salmon, P. (2004) Doctors' communication of trust, care and respect in breast cancer: qualitative study, *British Medical Journal*, 328(7444): 864.
Calnan, M. (1987) *Health and Illness: The Lay Perspective*. London: Tavistock Press.
Calnan, M. and Williams, S. (1992) Images of scientific medicine, *Sociology of Health and Illness*, 14(2): 233–54.
Calnan, M., Cant, S. and Gabe, J. (1993) *Going Private? The Use of Private Health Insurance*. Milton Keynes: Open University Press.
Calnan, M. and Ferlie, E. (2003) Analysing process in health care: the methodological and theoretical challenges, *Policy and Politics*, 131(2): 3–11.
Calnan, M., Montaner, D. and Horne, R. (2004) How acceptable are innovative health care technologies? A survey of public beliefs and attitudes in England and Wales, *Social Science and Medicine*, 60(9): 1937–948.
Calnan, M. and Rowe, R. (2004) *Trust in Health Care: An Agenda for Future Research*. London: The Nuffield Trust.

Calnan, M. and Rowe, R. (2006) Researching trust relations in health care: conceptual and methodological challenges, *Journal of Health Organisation and Management*, 20(5): 349–58.

Calnan, M. and Sanford, E. (2004) Public trust in health care: the system or the doctor? *Quality and Safety in Health Care*, 13: 92–97.

Calnan, M., Rowe, R. and Entwistle, V.A. (2006a) Trust relations in health care: an agenda for future research, *Journal of Health Organisation and Management*, 20(5): 477–84.

Calnan, M., Wainwright, D., Glasner, P., Newbury-Ecob, R. and Ferlie, E. (2006b) 'Medicine's next goldmine?' The implications of new genetic technologies, *Medicine, Health Care and Philosophy*, 9: 33–41.

Caress, A-L., Luker, K., Woodcock, A. and Beaver, K. (2002) A qualitative exploration of treatment decision-making role preference in adult asthma patients, *Health Expectations*, 5: 223–35.

Carr, G. (2001) Negotiating trust: a grounded theory study of inter-personal relationships between persons living with HIV/AIDS and their primary health care providers, *Journal of the Association of Nurses in Aids Care*, 12(2): 35–43.

Caterinicchio, R. (1979) Testing plausible path models of inter-personal trust in patient–physician treatment relationships, *Social Science and Medicine*, 13: 81–99.

Charles, C.A., Whelan, T., Gafni, A., Willan, A. and Farrell, S. (2003) Shared decision-making: what does it mean to physicians? *Journal of Clinical Oncology*, 21(5): 932–36.

Coburn, D., Rappolt, S. and Bourgeault, I. (1997) Decline vs retention of medical power through restratification: the Ontario case, *Sociology of Health and Illness*, 19: 1–22.

Collins, T., Clark, J., Patersen, L. and Kressin, N. (2002) Racial differences in how patients perceive physician communication regarding cardiac testing, *Medical Care*, 40(1): 127–34.

Connell, N.A.D. and Mannion, R. (2006) Conceptualisations of trust in the organisational literature: some indicators from a complementary perspective, *Journal of Health Organisation and Management*, 20(5): 417–33.

Cooper-Patrick, L., Powe, N., Gonzales, J., Levine, D. and Ford, D.E. (1997) Identification of patient attitudes and references regarding treatment for depression, *Journal of General Medicine*, 12: 431–38.

COSU (2002) *Risk*. London: Cabinet Office Strategy Unit.

Coulson, A. (1998) Trust and contract in public sector management, in A. Coulson (ed.) *Trust and Contracts: Relationships in Local Government Health and Public Services*. Bristol: Policy Press.

Darzi, A. (2007) *Our NHS Our Future NHS: Next Stage Review Interim Report*. London: The Stationery Office.

Davies, H.T.O. (1999) Falling public trust in health services: implications for accountability, *Journal of Health Service Research Policy*, 4(4): 193–94.

Davies, H.T.O. and Lampel, J. (1998) Trust in performance indicators, *Quality in Health Care*, 7: 159–62.

Davies, H.T.O. and Mannion, R. (2000) Clinical governance: striking a balance between checking and trusting, in P.C. Smith (ed.) *Reforming Markets in Health Care*. Milton Keynes: Open University Press.

Day, P. and Klein, R. (1987) *Accountabilities*. London: Tavistock Publications Ltd.

Degeling, P., Kennedy, J., Hill, M., Carnegie, M. and Holt, J. (1998) *Professional Sub-cultures and Hospital Reform*. University of New South Wales, Sydney: The Centre for Hospital Management and Information Systems Research.

Department of Health (1998) *A First Class Service: Quality in the New NHS*. London: The Stationery Office.

Department of Health (2002) *National Service Frameworks: A Practical Aid to Implementation in Primary Care*. London: The Stationery Office.

Department of Health (2003) *NHS Improvement Plan*. London: The Stationery Office.

Department of Health (2004a) *Choosing Health: Making Healthier Choices Easier*. London: The Stationery Office.

Department of Health (2004b) *Building on the Best: Choice, Responsiveness, and Equity in the NHS*. London: The Stationery Office.

Department of Health (2005) *Independence, Well-being and Choice: Our Vision for the Future of Social Care for Adults in England*. London: The Stationery Office.

Department of Health (2006) *Good Doctors, Safer Patients*. London: The Stationery Office.

Department of Health (2007) *Trust, Assurance and Safety: The Regulation of Health Professionals in the 21st Century*. London: The Stationery Office.

Dibben, M. and Lena, M. (2003) Achieving compliance in chronic illness management: illustrations of trust relationships between physicians and nutrition clinic patients, *Health, Risk and Society*, 5(3): 241–59.

Doescher, M.P. (2000) Racial and ethnic disparities in perceptions of physican style and trust, *Archives of Family Medicine*, 9: 1156–63.

Ellins, J. (2005) When know means know, *Health Service Journal*, 10 November: 24–25.

Entwistle, V.A. and Quick, O. (2006) Trust in the context of patient safety problems, *Journal of Health Organisation and Management*, 20(5): 397–416.

Evetts, J. (1999) Professionalisation and professionalism: issues for inter-professional care, *Journal of Interprofessional Care*, 13(2): 119–28.

Evetts, J. (2006) Introduction, trust and professionalism: challenges and occupational changes, *Current Sociology*, 54: 607–20.

Ferlie, E. and Geraghty, K.J. (2007) Professionals in public service organizations, in E. Ferlie, L.E. Lynn and C. Pollitt (eds) *The Oxford Handbook of Public Management*. Oxford: Oxford University Press.

Flynn, R. (2002) Clinical governance and governmentality, *Health, Risk and Society*, 4(2): 155–73.

Fox, A. (1974) *Beyond Contract: Work, Power and Trust Relations*. London: Faber.

Freburger, J.K., Callahan, L.F., Currey, S.S. and Anderson, L.A. (2003) Use of trust in physician scale in patients with rheumatic disease: psychometric properties and correlates of trust in the rheumatologist, *Arthritis and Rheumatism*, 49(1): 51–58.

Friedson, E. (1994) *Professionalism Reborn: Theory, Prophecy and Policy*. Cambridge: Polity Press.

Friedson, E. (2001) *Professionalism: The Third Logic*. Chicago: University of Chicago Press.

Gambetta, D. (1988) *Making and Breaking Co-operative Relations*. Oxford: Blackwell.

Gibson, D.E. (1990) What makes clients trust nurses, *Spinal Cord Injury Nursing*, 7(4): 81–85.

Giddens, A. (1990) *The Consequences of Modernity*. Cambridge: Polity Press.

Giddens, A. (1991) *Modernity and Self-identity: Self and Society in the Late Modern Age*. Cambridge: Polity Press.

Giddens, A. (1994) Living in a post-traditional society, in U. Beck, A. Giddens and S. Lash (eds) *Reflexive Modernization: Politics,*

Tradition and Aesthetics in the Modern Social Order. Cambridge: Polity Press.

Gilson, L. (2003) Trust and the development of health care as a social institution, *Social Science and Medicine*, 56: 1453–68.

Gilson, L. (2006) Trust and health care: theoretical perspectives and research needs, *Journal of Health Organisation and Management*, 20(5): 359–75.

Gilson, L., Palmer, N. and Schneider, H. (2005) Trust and health worker performance: exploring a conceptual framework using South African evidence, *Social Science and Medicine*, 61(7): 1418–29.

Goddard, M. and Mannion, R. (1998) From competition to co-operation: new economic relationships in the National Health Service, *Health Economics*, 7: 105–19.

Goold, S. and Klipp, G. (2002) Managed care members talk about trust, *Social Science and Medicine*, 54(6): 879–88.

Green, J. (2004) Is trust an under-researched component of health-care organisation? *British Medical Journal*, 329: 384.

Greener, I. (2003) Patient choice in the NHS: the view from economic sociology, *Social Theory and Health*, 1: 72–89.

Grumbach, K., Selby, J., Darnberg, C., Bindman, A., Quesenberry, C., Truman, A. and Uratsu, C. (1999) Resolving the gatekeeper conundrum: what patients value in primary care and referrals to specialists, *Journal of the American Medical Association*, 281(3): 261–66.

Haas, J., Phillips, K., Baker, L., Sonneborn, D. and McCulloch, C. (2003) Is the prevalence of gatekeeping in a community associated with individual trust in medical care? *Medical Care*, 41(5): 660–68.

Hall, M. (2006) Researching medical trust in the United States, *Journal of Health Organisation and Management*, 20(5): 456–68.

Hall, M., Dogan, E., Zheng, B. and Mishra, A. (2001) Trust in physicians and medical institutions. Does it matter? *Milbank Quarterly*, 79(4): 613–39.

Hall, M., Camacho, F., Dugan, E. and Balkrishnan, R. (2002) Trust in the medical profession: conceptual and measurement issues, *Health Services Research*, 37(5): 1419–32.

Hallas, D., Butz, A. and Gitterman, B. (2004) Attitudes and beliefs for effective pediatric nurse practitioner and physician collaboration, *Journal of Pediatric Health Care*, 18: 77–86.

Hardey, M. (1999) Doctor in the house: the internet as a source of lay health knowledge and the challenge to expertise, *Sociology of Health and Illness*, (21): 820–35.

Harrison, S. and Smith, C. (2004) Trust and moral motivation: redundant resources in health and social care? *Policy and Politics*, 32(3): 371–86.

Henman, M.J., Butow, P.N., Brown, R.F., Boyle, F. and Tattersall, M.H.N. (2002) Lay constructions of decision-making in cancer, *Psycho-Oncology*, 11: 295–306.

Hirshman, A.O. (1970) *Exit, Voice and Loyalty*. Cambridge, MA: Harvard University Press.

Hobson-West, P. (2007) Trusting blindly can be the biggest risk of all: organised resistance to childhood vaccination in the UK, *Sociology of Health and Illness*, 29(2): 198–215.

Horne, R., Weinman, J. and Hankins, M. (1999) The beliefs about medicines: questionnare and the development and evaluation of a new method for assessing the cognitive representation of medicine, *Psychology and Health*, 14: 1–27.

Hsu, J., Schmittdiel, J., Krupat, E., Stein, T., Thom, D., Fireman, B. and Selby, J. (2003) Patient choice: a randomised controlled trial of provider selection, *Journal of General Internal Medicine*, 18: 319–25.

Hunt, G. (1995) *Whistleblowing in the Health Service*. London: Edward Arnold.

Jackson, L., Putnam, W., Twohig, P., Burge, F., Nicol, K. and Cox, J. (2004) What has trust got to do with it? Cardiac risk reduction and family physicians' discussions of evidence-based recommendations, *Health Risk and Society*, 60(3): 239–55.

Joffe, S., Manocchia, M. and Weeks, J. (2003) What do patients value in their hospital care? An empirical perspective on autonomy centred bioethics, *Journal of Medical Ethics*, 29:103–8.

Johansson, E. and Winkvist, A. (2002) Trust and transparency in human encounters in tuberculosis control: lessons learned from Vietnam, *Qualitative Health Research*, 12(4): 473–91.

Jones, K. (1998) Trust, in *Routledge Encyclopaedia of Philosophy*. London: Routledge.

Kai, J. and Crosland, A. (2001) Perspectives of people with enduring mental health from a community-based qualitative study, *British Journal of General Practice*, 51: 730–37.

Kao, A., Green, D., Zaslavsky, A., Koplan, J. and Cleary, P. (1998a) The relationship between method of physician payment and patient trust, *Journal of the American Medical Association*, 280(19): 1708–714.

Kao, A., Green, O., Zaslavsky, A., Koplan, J. and Cleary, P. (1998b) Patients' trust in their physicians, *Journal of General Internal Medicine*, 13(10): 681–85.

Keating, N., Green, O., Kao, A., Gazmararian, J., Wu, V. and Cleary, P. (2002) How are patients' specific ambulatory care experiences related to trust, satisfaction, and considering changing physicians? *Journal of General Internal Medicine*, 17(1): 29–40.

Kehoe, S. and Ponting, J. (2003) Value importance and value congruence as determinants of trust in policy actors, *Social Science and Medicine*, 57: 1065–75.

Khodyakov, D. (2007) Trust as a process, *Sociology*, 41(1): 115–32.

Klein, R. (1996) *The New Politics of the NHS*. London: Longman Publishing Group.

Klein, R. (1998) Regulating the medical profession: doctors and the public interest, *Health Care UK*, 152–63.

Kraetschner, N., Sharpe, N., Urowitz, S. and Deber, R. (2004) How does trust affect patient preferences for participation in decision making? *Health Expectations*, 7(4): 271–3.

Krupat, E., Bell, R.A., Kravitz, R.L., Thom, D. and Azari, R. (2001) When physicians and patients think alike: patient-centred beliefs and their impact on satisfaction and trust, *Journal of Family Practice*, 50(12): 1057–62.

Kuhlmann, E. (2006) Traces of doubt and sources of trust: health professions in an uncertain society, *Current Sociology*, 54(4): 607–20.

Laschinger, H., Finegan, J., Shamian, J. and Casier S. (2000) Organisational trust and empowerment in restructured healthcare settings, *Journal of Nursing Administration*, 30(9): 413–25.

Lee-Treweek, G. (2002) Trust in complementary medicine: the case of cranial osteopathy, *The Sociological Review*, 50(1): 48–68.

Lewicki, R.J. and Bunker, B.B. (1996) Developing and maintaining trust in work relationships, in R.M. Kramer and T.R. Tyler (eds) *Trust in Organizations: Frontiers of Theory and Research*. Thousand Oaks, CA: Sage.

Lewis, J.D. and Weigert, A. (1985) Trust as a social reality, *Social Forces*, 63: 967–85.

Lings, P., Evans, P., Seamark, D., Seamark, C., Sweeney, K., Dixon, M. and Pereira Gray, D. (2003) The doctor–patient relationship in US primary care, *Journal of the Royal Society of Medicine*, 96: 180–84.

Luhmann, N. (1979) *Trust and Power*. Chichester: Wiley.

Lukoschek, P. (2003) African Americans' beliefs and attitudes regarding hypertension and its treatment: a qualitative study, *Journal of Health Care for the Poor and Underserved*, 14(4): 566–87.

Lupton, D. (1994) *Medicine as Culture: Illness Disease and the Body in Western Societies.* London: Sage.

Lupton, D. (1996) Your life in their hands: trust in the medical encounter, in V. James and J. Gabe (eds) *Health and the Sociology of Emotions.* Oxford: Blackwell.

Mainous, A., Baker, R., Love, M., Pereira Gray, D. and Gill, J. (2001) Continuity of care and trust in one's physician: evidence from primary care in the US and the UK, *Family Medicine*, 33(1): 22–27.

Mainous, A., Kern, D., Hainer, B., Kneuper-Hall, R., Stephens, J. and Geesey, M. (2004) The relationship between continuity of care and trust with stage of cancer at diagnosis, *Family Medicine*, 36(1): 35–39.

Mannion, R. and Goddard, M. (2003) Public disclosure of comparative clinical performance data: lessons from the Scottish experience, *Journal of Evaluation in Clinical Practice*, 9: 277–86.

Mannion, R. and Smith, P. (1996) Trust and reputation in community care: theory and evidence, in P. Anand and A. McGuire (eds) *Changes in Health Care: Reflections on the NHS Internal Market.* London: Macmillan.

Marshall, M.N., Shekelle, P.G., Leatherman, S. and Brook, R. (2000) What do we expect to gain from the public release of performance data? A review of the evidence, *Journal of the American Medical Association*, 283(1866): 1874.

Matthews, A., Sellergren, S., Manfredi, C. and Williams, M. (2002) Factors influencing medical information seeking among African American cancer patients, *Journal of Health Communication*, 7: 205–19.

Mayer, R.C., Davis, J.H. and Schoorman, F.D. (1995) An integrative model of organization trust, *Academy of Management Review*, 23: 438–58.

Maynard, A. and Bloor, K. (2003) Trust and performance management in the medical marketplace, *Journal of the Royal Society of Medicine*, 96: 532–39.

Mazor, K.M., Simon, S.R., Yood, R.A., Martinson, B.C., Gunter, M.J., Reed, G.W. and Gurwitz, J.H. (2004) Health plan members' views about disclosure of medical errors, *Annals of International Medicine*, 140: 409–18.

McAllister, D.J. (1995) Affect- and cognition-based trust as foundations for interpersonal co-operation in organizations, *Academy of Management Journal*, 38(1): 24–59.

McKay, J., Luborsky, L., Barber, J., Kabasakalian-McKay, R., Zorrilla, E. and Cacciola, J. (1997) Affiliative trust–mistrust and immunity in depressed patients receiving supportive–expressive psychotherapy, *Psychotherapy Research*, 7(3): 249–60.

McKneally, M. and Martin, D. (2000) An entrustment model of consent for surgical treatment of life-threatening illness: perspective of patients requiring esophagectomy, *Journal of Thoracic and Cardiovascular Surgery*, 120: 264–69.

Mead, N. and Bower, P. (2000) Patient-centredness: a conceptual framework and review of the empirical literature, *Social Science and Medicine*, 51: 1087–90.

Mechanic, D. and Schlesinger, M. (1996) The impact of managed care on patients' trust in medical care and their physicians, *Journal of the American Medical Association*, 275: 1693–97.

Mechanic, D. (1998) Functions and limits of trust in providing medical care, *Journal of Health Politics, Policy and Law*, 23(4): 661–86.

Mechanic, D. (2004) In my chosen doctor I trust, *British Medical Journal*, 329: 1413–19.

Mechanic, D. and Meyer, S. (2000) Concepts of trust among patients with serious illness, *Social Science and Medicine*, 51: 657–68.

Mishra A. (1996) Organizational responses to crisis: the centrality of trust, in R.M. Kramer and T.R. Tyler (eds) *Trust in Organizations: Frontiers of Theory and Research*. Thousand Oaks, CA: Sage.

Misztal, B (1996) *Trust in Modern Societies*. Cambridge: Polity Press.

Mosley-Williams, A., Lumley, M., Gillis, M., Leisen, J. and Guice, D. (2002) Barriers to treatment adherence among African American and white women with systemic lupus erythematosus, *Arthritis and Rheumatism*, 47(6): 630–38.

Murphy, J., Chang, H., Montgomery, J., Rogers, W. and Safran, D. (2001) The quality of physician–patient relationships: patients' experiences 1996–1999, *Journal of Family Practice*, 50(2): 123–29.

Nettleton, S., Burrows, R. and Watt, I. (2008) Regulating medical bodies? *Sociology of Health and Illness*, 30: 333–348.

NHSE (1999) *Clinical Governance*, HSC 1999/065. Leeds: NHS Executive.

Newman, J. (1998) The dynamics of trust, in A. Conlon (ed.) *Trust and Continuity: Relationships in Local Government, Health and Public Services*. Bristol: Policy Press.

Northouse, P.G. (1979) Interpersonal trust and empathy in nurse–nurse relationships, *Nursing Research*, 28(6): 365–68.

OECD (2001) *Citizens as partners.* Paris: OECD.

O'Neill, O. (2002) *A Question of Trust: BBC Reith Lectures 2002.* Cambridge: Cambridge University Press.

O'Neill, O. (2004) Accountability, trust and informed consent in medical practice and research, *Clinical Medicine*, 4: 269–76.

Paul, M. and Oyebode, F. (1999) Competence of voluntary psychiatric patients to give valid consent to neuroleptic medication, *Psychiatric Bulletin*, 23: 463–66.

Payne, R.L. and Clark, M.C. (2003) Dispositional and situational determinants of trust in two types of managers, *International Journal of Human Resource Management*, 14(1): 128–38.

Pollitt, C.J. (1993) Audit and accountability: the missing dimension? *Journal of the Royal Society of Medicine*, 36: 209–11.

Power, M. (1997) *The Audit Society: Rituals of Verification.* Oxford: Oxford University Press.

Prior, L. (2003) Belief, knowledge and expertise: the emergence of the lay expert in medical sociology, *Sociology of Health and Illness*, 25: 41–47.

Prior, L., Wood, F., Lewis, G. and Pill R. (2003) Stigma revisited: disclosure of emotional problems in primary care consultations in Wales, *Social Science and Medicine*, 56(10): 41–47.

Putnam, R. (2000) *Bowling Alone: The Collapse and Revival of American Community.* New York: Simon & Schuster.

Rempel, J.K., Holmes, J.G. and Zanna, M.D. (1975) Trust in close relationships, *Journal of Personality and Social Psychology*, 49: 95–112.

Repper, J., Ford, R. and Cooke, A. (1994) How can nurses build trusting relationships with people who have severe and long-term mental health problems? Experiences of case managers and their clients, *Journal of Advanced Nursing*, 19: 1096–104.

Ritchie, J. and Spencer, L (1994) Qualitative data analysis for applied policy research, in A. Bryman and R.G. Burgess (eds) *Analysing Qualitative Data.* London: Routledge.

Robb, N. and Greenhalgh, T. (2006) Conceptualisations of trust in the organisational literature: some indicators from a complementary perspective, *Journal of Health Organisation and Management*, 20(5): 417–33.

Rose, A., Peters, N., Shea, J.A. and Armstrong, K. (2004) Development and testing of the health care system distrust scale, *Journal of General Internal Medicine*, 19(1): 57–67.

Rose-Ackerman, S. (2001) Trust, honesty and corruption: reflection on the state-building process, *European Journal of Sociology*, 42(3): 526–70.

Rothstein, B. (1998) *Just Institutions Matter: The Moral and Political Logic of the Universal Welfare State.* Cambridge University Press: Cambridge.

Rowe, R. (2003) The roles of the lay member in primary care groups and trusts: do they enhance public accountability? *Dissertation Abstracts International: A – the Humanities and Social Sciences.* www.hsrc.ac.uk/Current_research/research_projects/public_trust.htm Rowe R. (30.11.2004) *Trust in health care: a systematic review.*

Rowe, R. and Calnan, M. (2006) Trust relations in health care: developing a theoretical framework for the 'new' NHS, *Journal of Health Organisation and Management*, 20(5): 376–96.

Rowland, M. (2004) Linking physicians pay to the quality of care – a major experiment in the UK, *New England Journal of Medicine*, 351:(14): 1448–53.

Safran, D., Taira, D., Rogers, W., Kosinski, M., Ware, J. and Tarlov, A. (1998) Linking primary care performance to outcomes of care, *Journal of Family Practice*, 47(3): 213–20.

Safran, D.G., Montgomery, J.E., Chang, H., Murphy, J. and Rogers, W. (2001) Switching doctors: predictors of voluntary disenrollment form a primary physician's practice, *Journal of Family Practice*, 50(2): 130–36.

Salter, B. (1999) Change in the governance of medicine and the politics of self-regulation, *Policy and Politics*, 27(2): 143–58.

Salter, B (2000) *Medical Regulation and Public Trust: An International Review.* London: King's Fund.

Scambler, G. and Britten, N. (2001) System, lifeworld and doctor–patient interaction: issues of trust in a changing world, in G. Scambler (ed.) *Habermas, Critical Theory and Health.* London: Routledge.

Schneider, E.C. and Lieberman, T. (2001) Publicly disclosed information about the quality of health care: response of the US public, *Quality in Health Care*, 10: 96–103.

Schulz, R.I. and Harrison, S. (1986) Physician autonomy in the Federal Republic of Germany, Great Britain and the United States, *International Journal of Health Planning and Management*, 1(5): 1213–28.

Sharma, R., Haas, M. and Stano, M. (2003) Patient attitudes, insurance and other determinants of self-referral to medical and chiropractic physicians, *American Journal of Public Health*, 19(12): 2111–17.

Sharma, U. (1995) Using complementary therapies: a challenge to orthodox medicine? in S. Williams and M. Calnan (eds) *Modern Medicine: Lay Perspectives and Experiences*. London: UCL Press.

Sheaff, R., Schofield, J., Mannion, R., Dowling, B., Marshall, M. and McNally, R. (2004) *Organisational Factors and Performance: A Review of the Literature*. London: NHS Service Delivery and Organisational R&D Programme.

Skinner, T.C. and Hampson, S.E. (2001) Personal models of diabetes in relation to self-care, well-being, and glycemic control, *Diabetes Care*, 24(5): 828–33.

Smith, R. (1992) The GMC on performance: professional self-regulation is on the line, *British Medical Journal*, 304: 1257.

Smith, C. (2001) Trust and confidence: possibilities for social work in 'high modernity', *British Journal of Social Work*, 31: 287–305.

Sobo, E. (2001) Rationalization of medical risk through talk of trust an explanation of elective eye surgery narratives, *Anthropology and Medicine*, 8(2/3): 265–78.

Stapleton, H., Kirkham, M. and Thomas, G. (2002) Qualitative study of evidence-based leaflets in maternity care, *British Medical Journal*, 324: 639.

Stevenson, F. and Scambler, G. (2005) The relationship between medicine and the public: the challenge of concordance, *Health*, 9(1): 5–21.

Stewart, M. and Roter, D. (1989) *Communicating with Medical Patients*, London: Sage.

Straten, G., Friele, R. and Groenewegen, D. (2002) Public trust in health care, *Social Science and Medicine*, 55: 227–34.

Strauss, A. and Corbin J. (1998) *Basics of Qualitative Research*. Thousand Oaks, CA: Sage.

Sulmasy, D., Bloche, M., Mitchell, J. and Hadley J. (2000) Physicians' ethical beliefs about cost-control arrangements, *Archives of Internal Medicine*, 160: 649–57.

Svedberg, P., Jormfeldt, H. and Arvidsson, B. (2003) Patients' conceptions of low health processes are promoted in mental health nursing, *Journal of Psychiatric and Mental Health Nursing*, 10(4): 448–56.

Sztompka, P. (1999) *Trust: A Sociological Theory*. Cambridge: Cambridge University Press.

Tarrant, C., Stokes, T. and Baker, R. (2003) Factors associated with patients' trust in their general practitioner: a cross-sectional survey, *British Journal of General Practice*, 53: 798–800.

Taylor, D. and Bury, M. (2007) Chronic illness, expert patients and care transition, *Sociology of Health and Illness*, 29(1): 127–45.

Taylor, G. (1998) Underperforming doctors: a postal survey of the Northern Deanery, *British Medical Journal*, 316: 1705–8.

Taylor-Gooby, P. (2008) Trust and welfare state reform: the example of the NHS, *Social Policy and Administration*, 42, 3: 288–306.

Taylor-Gooby, P. and Hastie, C. (2003) Paying for world class services: a British dilemma, *Journal of Social Policy*, 32(2): 271–88.

Taylor, R., Pringle, M. and Coupland, C. (2004) *Implications of Offering 'Patient Choice' for Routine Adult Surgical Referrals*. London: Dr Foster Ltd.

Thom, D., Hall, M. and Pawlson, L. (2004) Measuring patients' trust in their physicians when assessing quality of care, *Health Affairs*, 23(4): 124–32.

Thom, D. and Ribisi, K. (1999) Further validation and reliability testing of the trust in physician scale, *Medical Care*, 37(5): 510–517.

Thom, D.H., Ribisl, K.M., Stewart, A.L. and Luke, D.A. (1999) Further validation and reliability testing of the trust in physician scale, *Medical Care*, 37(5): 510–17.

Thom, D.H., Kravitz, R.L., Bell, R.A., Krupat, E. and Azari, R. (2002) Patient trust in the physician: relationship to patient requests, *Family Practice*, 19: 476–83.

Thorne, S.E. and Robinson, C.A. (1988) Health care relationships: the chronic illness perspective, *Research in Nursing & Health*, 11: 293–300.

Thorne, S.E. and Robinson, C.A. (1989) Guarded alliance: health care relationships in chronic illness, *Journal of Nursing Scholarship*, 21(3): 153–57.

Titmuss, R. (1968) *Commitment to Welfare*. London: George Allen & Unwin Ltd.

Titmuss, R. (1987) Choice and the welfare state, in B. Abel-Smith and K.C. Titmuss (eds) *The Philosophy of Welfare*. London: Allen & Unwin.

Trojan, L. and Yonge, O. (2003) Developing trusting, caring relationships: home care nurses and elderly clients, *Journal of Advanced Nursing*, 8: 1903–910.

Tyler, T.R. and Kramer, R.M. (1996) Whither trust? in R.M. Kramer and T.R. Tyler (eds) *Trust in Organizations: Frontiers of Theory and Research*. London: Sage.

van der Schee, E., Braun, B., Calnan, M., Schnee, M. and Groenewegen, D. (2003) Public trust in health care: a comparison of Germany, the Netherlands, and England and Wales, *European Journal of Public Health*, 13(4): 78.

van der Schee, E., Groenewegen, P. and Friele, R. (2006) Public trust in health care: a performance indicator? *Journal of Health Organisation and Management*, 20(5): 468–76.

van der Schee, E., Braun, B., Calnan, M., Schnee, M. and Groenewegen, D. (2007) Public trust in health care: a comparison of Germany, The Netherlands, and England and Wales, *Health Policy*, 81: 56–67.

Walker, J. and Brooksby, M. (1998) Patient perceptions of hospital care: building confidence, *Journal of Nursing Management*, 6(4): 193–200.

Warren, M.E. (1999) *Democracy and Trust*. Cambridge: Cambridge University Press.

Williams, S. and Calnan, M. (1996) Conclusions; modern medicine and the lay populace in late modernity, in S. Williams and M. Calnan (eds) *Modern Medicine: Lay Perspectives and Experiences*. London: UCL Press.

Wilson, S., Morse, J.M. and Penrod, J. (1998) Developing reciprocal trust in the care-giving relationship, *Qualitative Health Research*, 8(4): 446–65.

Zadoroznyj, M. (2001) Birth and the 'reflexive consumer': trust, risk and medical dominance in obstetric encounters, *Journal of Sociology*, 37(2): 117–39.

Zinn, J.O. and Taylor-Gooby, P. (2006) Risk as an interdisciplinary research area, in P. Taylor-Gooby and J.O. Zinn (eds) *Risk in Social Science*. Oxford: Oxford University Press.

Zucker, L.G. (1986) Production of trust: institutional sources of economic structure 1840–1920, in B.M. Staw and L.L. Cummings (eds) *Research in Organizational Behaviour*. Greenwich, CT: JAI Press.

INDEX

Locators shown in *italics* refer to figures and tables.

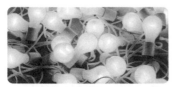 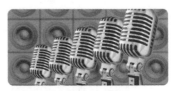
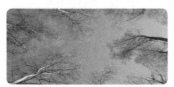 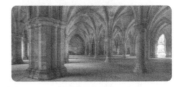
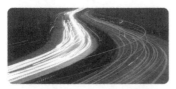 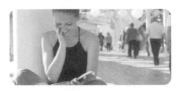
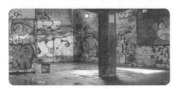
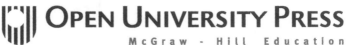